Unstable angina and non-Q-wave myocardial infarction

Derek Waller
Consultant Cardiovascular Phy[...]
Southampton General Hospital
Southampton SO16 6YD

Introduction

Unstable angina and non-Q-wave myocardial infarction (MI) are part of the spectrum of ischaemic heart disease ranging from stable angina to full thickness or Q-wave MI. Unstable angina is a clinical syndrome, which often, but not always, involves ischaemic pain at rest. There are three distinct patient groups:

Those with new onset angina of effort, especially when severe;

Those with abrupt increase in the frequency, severity, or duration of pre-existing stable angina; *and*

Those developing angina within one month after MI.

Non-Q-wave MI usually presents as prolonged ischaemic chest pain, associated with a rise in cardiac enzymes, but without Q-waves on the ECG.

In both unstable angina and non-Q-wave infarction, electrocardiogram (ECG) changes may be present, including ST-segment elevation or depression and T-wave inversion, but in unstable angina the ECG may be normal or show only transient changes, even during the pain. If the activity of plasma myocardial enzymes eg, creatine kinase is raised to more than twice the upper limit of normal, the patient has suffered a MI. However, lesser enzyme increases can occur in unstable angina. In particular, more sensitive enzymatic markers of myocardial damage, eg, troponin I or T, are raised in up to one-third of patients with acute coronary syndromes who have normal plasma creatine kinase activity[1].

MI presenting with ST-segment elevation on the ECG carries the highest mortality risk in the subsequent 30 days. However, both non-Q-wave infarction (with or without ST-segment elevation) and unstable angina carry an 8-15% risk of death in the subsequent four months, with a similar risk of non-fatal MI. After this time, the risk is similar to that in stable angina.

Two-thirds of patients with chest pain presenting to an Accident and Emergency Department do not have an acute coronary syndrome. An accurate history is important for reaching a diagnosis, but the use of an ECG and enzymes such as troponin I or T can help in the initial triage of these patients into high- and low-risk categories for a subsequent ischaemic event[2].

Pathophysiology
Most acute coronary syndromes are caused by unstable atheromatous plaques. The most vulnerable plaques are those with a lipid-rich core and a thin fibrous cap. Fissuring or erosion of such a plaque, which might itself cause only mild or moderate obstruction, promotes thrombus formation. The resulting ischaemic syndrome is determined by the extent and duration of the occlusion of the artery. Unstable angina arises if the thrombus is non-occlusive and a non-Q-wave infarction follows an occlusive thrombus with early subsequent reperfusion.

Unstable angina can also arise from coronary vasoconstriction, usually occurring at the site of an atheromatous plaque. Common precipitants of vasospasm include cold, emotional stress, or release of vasoconstrictors from local platelet thrombus.

In some patients, unstable symptoms can arise from potentially treatable exacerbating conditions, eg, uncontrolled hypertension, persistent sinus tachycardia or another arrhythmia, thyrotoxicosis or anaemia.

Management

Unfortunately, in many patients with acute coronary syndromes the diagnosis is not made until the condition has progressed to a Q-wave MI. Early treatment can reduce the risk of progression and may also reduce mortality. However, not all patients are at the same risk of ischaemic complications in the days immediately after the onset of unstable symptoms. Early predictors of higher risk of complications in the subsequent few days include:

Ischaemic pain at rest lasting more than 20 minutes;

ST-segment elevation or depression on the ECG of more than 1 mm (particularly in the anterior chest leads) in association with rest pain; *and*

Angina accompanied by signs of left ventricular failure or hypotension.

The immediate management of patients with a suspected acute coronary syndrome depends on the clinical circumstances. If the symptoms or ECG suggest a high risk of complications immediate admission to hospital should be arranged. If the patient is not taking aspirin regularly, a 300 mg loading dose should be given either as soluble aspirin, or as a standard tablet, chewed before swallowing, for a rapid onset of its antiplatelet effect. Sublingual glyceryl trinitrate should be tried for all patients in pain, and oxygen is often given, although evidence for its value is lacking. If rest pain is absent and the symptoms are not rapidly progressive, treatment with an antianginal agent and aspirin may be sufficient, without immediate hospital admission, provided arrangements are made for urgent outpatient assessment by a cardiovascular physician.

The aims of treatment of all acute coronary syndromes are to relieve symptoms and reduce the risk of a subsequent, more serious event.

Medical management controls symptoms in about 90% of patients with unstable angina requiring hospital admission[3].

Antiplatelet agents
Aspirin is the drug of choice, and is effective at a dosage of 75 mg daily after an initial 300 mg loading dose. In the Antiplatelet Triallists Collaboration report, aspirin reduced the vascular event rate in unstable angina from 14% to 9%[4]. Similar results have been reported for aspirin in acute MI. If aspirin is contraindicated or not tolerated, clopidogrel, an inhibitor of ADP-mediated platelet aggregation, could be considered. There are no data for this drug in unstable angina and it is not licensed for this indication, but it shows similar efficacy to aspirin in preventing recurrent stroke or MI[5].

The most exciting development in antiplatelet therapy is the use of the powerful glycoprotein 11b/111a inhibitors, such as tyrofiban. Several trials with these drugs in unstable angina have reported reductions in a composite endpoint of death, MI and the need for emergency revascularisation, particularly when used in combination with heparin. However, the additional benefits are small, most marked during the period of treatment, and decline with time[6]. It is likely that these drugs will only be cost-effective in the small group of high-risk patients, particularly those with raised plasma troponin I or T concentrations.

Anticoagulants
Trials of intravenous unfractionated heparin alone in unstable angina have produced inconsistent results, but heparin is beneficial when used with aspirin. Meta-analysis of the intervention trials shows, that compared with aspirin alone, the combination reduces the risk of MI or death by 33% (an absolute risk reduction from 10.4% with aspirin alone to 7.9%)[7]. The optimal duration of treatment with heparin is uncertain, but giving it for 48 hours may maximise benefit and minimise the risk of bleeding[8].

More recently, low molecular weight (LMW) heparin has been compared with unfractionated heparin, both in combination with aspirin.

LMW heparin can be given by subcutaneous injection and does not require routine monitoring of its anticoagulant effect, giving it the potential advantage of ease of use. Published trials have used enoxaparin or dalteparin for between two and eight days in patients with unstable angina or non-Q-wave infarction. LMW heparin was either similar to, or marginally better than, unfractionated heparin for reducing death, MI or recurrent angina[6]. The optimal dosage regimen and duration of treatment with LMW heparin are unknown. At present, therefore, the decision to use LMW heparin rather than unfractionated heparin must rest on whether its ease of use offsets the additional cost.

There is some concern that short-term use of heparin may be followed by a rebound increase in ischaemic events when it is stopped. Prolonging treatment with subcutaneous heparin or warfarin for six to twelve weeks may reduce this risk, but definitive evidence is lacking.

Thrombolysis
Although the pathophysiological mechanism of unstable angina is similar to that of MI, thrombolysis with streptokinase or tissue plasminogen activator has consistently failed to show any benefit. Overall, thrombolysis is associated with a small increase in mortality.

Antianginal drugs
Beta-adrenoceptor antagonists are the first-line antianginal treatment for unstable angina if there are no contraindications. A meta-analysis of studies with various beta-blockers indicated a 13% reduction in subsequent MI[9]. In patients with rest pain or those at high risk, an initial intravenous dose (eg, atenolol, 5 mg then a further 5 mg after ten minutes) should be given. Oral treatment is adequate for lower risk patients. If beta-blockade is contraindicated then oral diltiazem can be considered, based on extrapolation from the results of intravenous use[10].

Nitrates are widely used for treatment of unstable angina, and can be very effective for symptom relief. Surprisingly, there are no randomised placebo-controlled trials of the effect of nitrates on either symptoms or cardiac events. Glyceryl trinitrate should be given sublingually (up to 1.5 mg) or buccally (initially 3 mg, increasing rapidly until pain control is achieved) to all patients with symptoms suggestive of unstable angina who have continuing pain. Intravenous glyceryl trinitrate (initially 5-10 micrograms per minute), or isosorbide dinitrate, can be given if the pain is not relieved. Dosage titration can be carried out at ten-minute intervals until symptoms are relieved or excessive hypotension ensues (systolic blood pressure <90 mmHg, or more than a 30% fall if there is significant pre-treatment hypertension). After the symptoms have been stabilised, oral nitrate therapy can be substituted, using a regimen that gives a nitrate-free or nitrate-low period to minimise the development of tolerance.

Nifedipine and related calcium antagonists should not be used alone in unstable angina. Trials with short-acting nifedipine suggested a trend to an increased risk of MI or recurrent ischaemia. However, when nifedipine is added to beta-blockade for patients with continuing pain, symptom relief is improved[11]. The potassium-channel opener nicorandil was recently shown to produce symptomatic benefit in patients whose pain is uncontrolled by maximal dosages of other antianginal agents[12].

Coronary angiography

Invasive investigation, with a view to revascularisation, should be considered for all patients with recurrent episodes of myocardial ischaemia despite maximal medical therapy. Other high-risk patient groups who should be considered for angiography after symptoms have settled include those with ST-segment changes on the ECG during pain, those with an exercise test showing ischaemic change and those with a raised troponin I or T concentration at the time of the acute episode[13,14]. Routine early invasive investigation with subsequent coronary angioplasty or bypass surgery carries no prognostic advantage, and some studies have shown a detrimental effect of such a strategy on subsequent ischaemic events. If possible, the symptoms should be controlled with medical therapy before more invasive investigation.

Lipid-lowering therapy

There is substantial evidence supporting the use of lipid-lowering therapy, particularly statins, in patients following acute coronary syndromes. Most studies have addressed the management of patients after MI (eg, 4S, CARE[15,16]) but the more recent LIPID study demonstrated similar long-term benefit after an episode of unstable angina[17]. Based on these studies, the ideal plasma total cholesterol concentration after an episode of unstable angina or a non-Q-wave infarction should be below 5.0 mmol/L, at least in patients below the age of 75 years.

Other measures

Management should, where appropriate, include advice on smoking cessation, dietary modification, weight loss, control of diabetes, control of hypertension, and an increase in exercise, as is the case with all other syndromes of coronary artery disease.

Conclusions

- Unstable angina and non-Q-wave infarction carry a high risk of subsequent ischaemic events.
- Immediate admission to hospital is advisable for patients with rest pain.
- Aspirin and heparin used concurrently reduce the risk of subsequent MI.
- Nitrates relieve symptoms but their effect on outcome is unknown. In the absence of contraindications, a beta-blocker is the antianginal agent of choice.
- Angiography may be desirable once symptoms have settled if there is a raised plasma troponin I or T concentration in the first eight hours after the onset of symptoms, or an exercise test is positive once symptoms have settled.
- In the long-term, attention to risk factors, especially plasma cholesterol, will reduce event rates.

References

1. Rottbauer W, Greten T, Muller-Bardorff M et al. Troponin T: a marker for myocardial infarction and minor cardiac cell damage. *Eur Heart J* 1996; **17 (suppl F):** 3-8.

2. Roberts R, Fromm RE. Management of acute coronary syndromes based on risk stratification by biochemical markers: an idea whose time has come. *Circulation* 1998; **98:** 1831-3.

3. Conti CR, Hill JA, Mayfield WR. Unstable angina pectoris: pathogenesis and management. *Curr Prob Cardiol* 1989; **14:** 549-624.

4. Antiplatelet Triallists Collaboration. Collaborative overview of randomized trials of antiplatelet therapy - I: Prevention of death, myocardial infarction, and stroke by prolonged antiplatelet therapy in various categories of patients. *BMJ* 1994; **308:** 81-106.

5. CAPRIE Steering Committee. A randomised, blinded, trial of clopidogrel versus aspirin in patients at risk of ischaemic events (CAPRIE). *Lancet* 1996; **348:** 1329-39.

6. Steeds RP, Channer KS. Recent advances in the management of unstable angina and non-Q-wave myocardial infarction. *Br J Clin Pharmacol* 1998; **46:** 335-41.

7. Oler A, Whooley MA, Oler J, Grady D. Adding heparin to aspirin reduces the incidence of myocardial infarction in death in patients with unstable angina. A meta-analysis. *JAMA* 1996; **276:** 811-5.

8. Klein LW, Wahid F, VandenBerg BJ, Parillo JE, Calvin JE. Comparison of heparin therapy for < or = 48 hours and >48 hours in unstable angina pectoris. *Am J Cardiol* 1997; **79:** 259-63.

9. Yusuf S, Wittes J, Friedman L. Overview of results of randomized clinical trials in heart disease. II. Unstable angina, heart failure, primary prevention with aspirin and risk factor modification. *JAMA* 1988; **260:** 2259-63.

10. Gobel EJ, van Gilst WH, de Kam PJ, ter Napel MG, Molhoek GP, Lie KI. Long-term follow-up after early intervention with intravenous diltiazem or intravenous nitroglycerine for unstable angina pectoris. *Eur Heart J* 1998; **19:** 1208-13.

11. Held PH, Yusuf S, Furberg CD. Calcium channel blockers in acute myocardial infarction and unstable angina: an overview. *BMJ* 1989; **299:** 1187-92.

12. Patel DJ, Purcell HJ, Fox KM. Cardioprotection by opening of the K(ATP) channel in unstable angina. Is this a clinical manifestation of myocardial preconditioning? Results of a randomized study with nicorandil. CESAR 2 investigation. Clinical European studies in angina and revascularization. *Eur Heart J* 1999; **20:** 51-7.

13. Newby LK, Christenson RH, Ohman M, et al. Value of serial troponin T measures for early and late risk stratification in patients with acute coronary syndromes. The GUSTO-IIa Investigators. *Circulation* 1998; **98:** 853-9.

14. Lindhl B, Andren B, Ohlsson J, Venge P, Wallentin L. Risk stratification in unstable coronary artery disease. Additive value of troponin T determinations and pre-discharge exercise tests. FRISK Study Group. *Eur Heart J* 1997; **18:** 762-70.

15. The Scandinavian Simvastatin Survival Study Group. Randomised trial of cholesterol lowering in 4444 patients with coronary heart disease: the Scandinavian Simvastatin Survival Study (4S). *Lancet* 1994; **344:** 1383-9.

16. Sacks FM, Pfeffer MA, Moye LA, et al. The effect of pravastatin on coronary events after myocardial infarction in patients with average cholesterol levels. Cholesterol and Resurrent Events Trial investigators. *N Engl J Med* 1996; **335:** 1001-9.

17. The Long-Term Intervention with Pravastatin in Ischaemic Disease (LIPID) Study Group. Prevention of cardiovascular events and death with pravastatin in patients with coronary heart disease and a broad range of initial cholesterol levels. *N Engl J Med* 1998; **339:** 1349-57.

Hypercholesterolaemia: primary prevention

Paul Durrington
Professor of Medicine
University of Manchester
Department of Medicine
Manchester Royal Infirmary
Manchester M13 9WL

Introduction

The incidence of coronary heart disease (CHD) is very high in the United Kingdom (UK), but elsewhere in the world it is often much lower. Epidemiological studies show a strong correlation between the average serum cholesterol of a population and its rate of CHD. Differences in average cholesterol concentrations probably relate to the proportion of dietary energy derived from carbohydrates as opposed to fat, particularly saturated fat, and rates of obesity. Cigarette smoking, hypertension and diabetes mellitus, although important determinants of CHD risk in high-cholesterol societies such as Britain, have less impact on it in countries whose populations have low serum cholesterol levels. Despite this, until recently British recommendations for CHD prevention tended to assume that the role of cholesterol is minor and simply advise a population strategy based on nutritional change, without the need for its clinical diagnosis and management based on individual risk. However there is good evidence that specific groups benefit from drug therapy to decrease serum cholesterol, both in terms of decreased CHD risk and overall mortality[1-5].

Screening

Selection of patients for intervention should not be based on single risk-factors in isolation, eg, high blood pressure or high cholesterol, but rather on detection of patients at high cardiovascular risk who will benefit most from intervention. Although this risk may be the consequence of a considerable increase in one factor as in, for example, accelerated hypertension or familial hypercholesterolaemia, it is more commonly the consequence of the combined effect of increases in several factors which would not increase the risk enough to require drug therapy were they isolated phenomena.

More direct evidence is needed of the benefit, possible harm, population cost and individual cost-effectiveness of routine population screening followed by drug treatment of hyperlipidaemia or hypertension. Nevertheless, in the meantime, clinicians need a method of ensuring that drug treatment is directed to those most likely to benefit. My personal approach is to advise screening of everyone above an age when high cardiovascular risk is detectable in a significant proportion of the population, which probably means after the age of 40 years. There is also undoubtedly a case for measuring cholesterol by the age of five years, in those where familial hypercholesterolaemia is either possible because of a definite diagnosis in a parent or sibling, or the suspected diagnosis in a parent who has died prematurely[6]. On the other hand, including people over the age of 70 years in general population screening will yield a very large proportion at high risk, for whom there is much less evidence of benefit from treatment. There is also no point in screening unless a clear management plan has been decided on for patients above a certain level of risk, and adequate arrangements have been made to monitor patients whose level of risk is borderline for treatment, but likely to increase to a level where active intervention is justified in future.

Although the incidence of CHD is higher in men of all ages, it is also a major cause of morbidity and death in women, and there is no evidence that women do not derive as much benefit from interventions. Because of their lower average cardiovascular risk, screening in women might reasonably, however, begin later than in men, probably around the age of 50 years. Hormone replacement therapy (HRT) should not be considered an adequate means of preventing CHD in women. The observational evidence relating to HRT is of lower quality than the evidence of benefit from cholesterol- and blood pressure-lowering drugs in placebo-controlled trials and the first placebo-controlled trial of HRT in women with established CHD failed to show any evidence of benefit[7].

The degree of risk to seek in screening depends on the level at which intervention is considered appropriate. In view of the relative freedom from major side-effects of statin and antihypertensive therapy, this is - to a large extent - determined by the cost of therapy and the medical and nursing manpower available to monitor treatment. The recently published joint recommendations of the British Cardiac Society (BCS), British Hyperlipidaemia Association (BHA) and the British Hypertension Society (BHS)[8] endorse the earlier Standing Medical Advisory Committee (SMAC) guidelines[9] that patients without known CHD or other major atherosclerotic disease should receive statin therapy, if their CHD risk is 3% annually, or greater. However, this was considered the current minimum acceptable standard of care and the guidelines proposed that we should eventually aim to treat patients at 1.5% or greater annual CHD risk. Already several European learned societies with an interest in cardiovascular disease recommend that statins should be prescribed in primary prevention when CHD risk exceeds 2% annually[10]. The problem of cost with statin therapy is not simply the price of the drugs, but the sheer scale of the number of people who could benefit from them in Britain.

The joint BCS/BHA/BHS recommendations are to begin statin therapy for primary prevention in patients above the threshold risk with cholesterol concentrations >5 mmol/L. The risk of future CHD events in some candidates for primary prevention overlaps with that of patients with established CHD and it is logical to use the same cholesterol threshold in both groups.

Risk assessment
Whatever level of CHD risk is targeted in primary prevention, the clinician requires a more accurate method of risk assessment than

relying entirely on clinical judgement. As the most comprehensive set of risk-factors incorporated in a mathematical equation predicting CHD risk in both men and women is that derived from the Framingham Study[11], virtually all of the major recommendations about CHD prevention are based on predictions from this equation. The weakness is that these data were taken from an unrepresentative volunteer population from a single United States (US) town many years ago and may not be applicable to the British population, but in men at least there was agreement between the Framingham equation and events in the West of Scotland Coronary Prevention Study[12]. An equation for both men and women based on British data would be welcome.

Current US and European guidelines, based on the Framingham equation, use either an algorithm to determine which patients should receive cholesterol-lowering therapy[13] or a chart to estimate individual risk[10]. In Britain, the Sheffield Risk & Treatment Table, also derived from the Framingham equation, was recommended by SMAC to identify people at a CHD event risk greater than 3% annually[14]. Methods such as these, based on total cholesterol alone, are less accurate than those based on the full Framingham equation as they assume the same mean high-density lipoprotein (HDL) value for all subjects[15]. Patients suspected of being at high CHD risk should have both HDL cholesterol and total serum cholesterol measured, for which the patient need not fast.

The joint British guidelines[8] are accompanied by a computer programme, which includes HDL cholesterol and allows the clinician to predict a patient's risk of CHD and stroke as a percentage over 10 years. A knowledge of stroke risk can be important in deciding when to treat mild hypertension. The joint British guidelines also provide a chart which allows practitioners without access to a computer in their consulting rooms to predict CHD risk. By way of illustration, one section of the chart is shown in Figure 1.

Certain patients are at higher risk than predicted by the Framingham equation, eg, those with proteinuria, patients with insulin-dependent

Figure 1

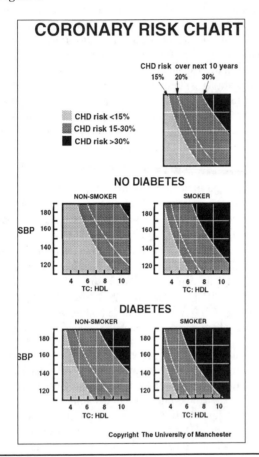

CHD= Coronary heart disease, SBP = Systolic blood pressure, TC = Total cholesterol, HDL = High-density lipoprotein

diabetes mellitus (in whom HDL cholesterol levels tend to be high, but who are still at high risk of vascular disease), British Asians, patients with a family history of premature CHD and with familial hypercholesterolaemia. Left ventricular hypertrophy also increases risk, yet is frequently omitted from risk prediction charts.

Raised triglycerides

Every patient who is being seriously considered for statin therapy should have a fasting biochemical evaluation, including triglycerides. This excludes patients with markedly raised triglycerides (>5 mmol/L), for whom statin therapy may not be appropriate, and who may require specialist evaluation. A retrospective analysis of clinical trial results indicates that drugs lowering both cholesterol and serum triglycerides may have a greater effect on CHD risk than might be expected from cholesterol reduction alone[16]. Triglycerides are an independent risk-factor for CHD[17], but are not included in the Framingham equation in which probably much of their influence as a risk factor is assigned to HDL. Clinicians should be aware that patients with raised triglycerides are likely to be at higher risk than similar patients with lower levels of triglycerides.

Age

There was no suggestion in the statin trials that the relative decrease in CHD incidence was attenuated by age although patients were only recruited into the trials up to the age of 75 years. Because the absolute risk of CHD increases with age, a larger proportion of a treated elderly population stand to benefit than in younger age groups. The reason for restricting statin treatment according to age is based on considerations such as cost and quality of life rather than scientific evidence of lack of efficacy or increased adverse effects. The present recommendation is that the upper age limit for initiating lipid-lowering medication for primary prevention should be 69 years.

Diet

There is evidence that dietary advice (as opposed to a diet administered on a metabolic ward, in elemental form or to trained volunteers) is not an effective means of lowering cholesterol. A recent appraisal of dietary trials has shown that overall, the best that can be achieved is a reduction in total cholesterol of about 5%[18], much less than the 20% achieved in the statin trials. Evidence that supplementing the diet with polyunsaturates reduces CHD is stronger than that for simple reduction of saturated fat[19]. However, general dietary advice to lose weight and to decrease saturated fat intake should not be abandoned. In lean individuals, any energy deficiency can be made up from mono-unsaturated or polyunsaturated fatty acids, especially from oily fish, and patients need not go to the expense of buying olive oil, because rapeseed oil is very similar in composition and considerably cheaper. There is no clinical trial evidence that antioxidants are effective in primary CHD prevention. The essential point is that diet should be seen as an adjunct to statin therapy and not a substitute for it.

The choice of statin

Pravastatin in a dose of 40 mg has been shown to be safe and effective in reducing CHD incidents in both primary[1] and secondary[4,5] prevention. Similar evidence is available for lovastatin (not licensed in the UK) in primary prevention[2] and for simvastatin in secondary prevention[3]. Based on the trial evidence pravastatin in a dose of 40 mg daily should thus be the drug of first choice in primary CHD prevention in Britain. Simvastatin may be used in patients intolerant of pravastatin or who do not achieve their target cholesterol level (see later) on pravastatin 40 mg daily. The cost of both pravastatin and simvastatin has recently been reduced so that for both the prices of 20 mg and 40 mg are the same (£380 annually), substantially less than the £550 annually for simvastatin in the dose employed in 4S[3] used in earlier calculation of cost-effectiveness[14]. Further savings can only be made by prescribing pravastatin or simvastatin in daily doses of 10 mg or by accepting both the benefit and safety of statins as class effects, in which case atorvastatin and cerivastatin are cheaper for an equivalent degree of cholesterol lowering. For patients with markedly elevated cholesterol, for example those with familial hypercholesterolaemia, atorvastatin is the most efficacious in reducing cholesterol and can be used in daily doses of up to 80 mg.

The aim of statin therapy

The statin trials used either a fixed dose of drug, a treatment target based on the total cholesterol or one based on LDL cholesterol, and all produced similar relative reductions in CHD. It therefore seems most practical and economical to base the target of treatment on the total cholesterol concentration and to titrate the dose of statin to reduce this below 5.0 mmol/L. For clinicians whose laboratories routinely report the low-density lipoprotein (LDL), or who wish to calculate this using the Friedwald equation, the equivalent LDL target is 3.0 mmol/L. In patients whose serum cholesterol is relatively low before statin treatment is initiated (5-6 mmol/L) a decrease of 30% may be a more logical aim of therapy. As discontinuing statin therapy usually results in an increase in serum cholesterol to pre-treatment levels or more within about one month, treatment should generally be regarded as lifelong.

Conclusions

- Screening should be for CHD risk as a whole, not for individual risk factors such as raised blood pressure or raised cholesterol.
- Serum and HDL cholesterol should be part of a risk assessment, but neither of these measurements need be made in the fasting state.
- Clinical assessment of risk should not be based on clinical judgement alone: it is improved by the use of a computer programme or a chart.
- Statins are indicated now in primary prevention of CHD when annual CHD risk is >3% and, when and where resources allow, >1.5%.
- Dietary advice should not be regarded either as unimportant or as an alternative to statin therapy in high risk patients. It does, however, require re-evaluation.

References

1. Shepherd J, Cobbe SM, Ford I, et al. Prevention of coronary heart disease with pravastatin in men with hypercholesterolaemia. West of Scotland Coronary Prevention Group. *N Engl J Med* 1995; **333:** 1301-7.

2. Downs GR, Clearfield M, Weiss S, et al. Primary prevention of acute coronary events with lovastatin in men and women with average cholesterol levels: results of the AFCAPS/TexCAPS. Air Force/Texas Coronary Atherosclerosis Prevention Study. *JAMA* 1998; **279:** 1615-22.

3. Scandinavian Simvastatin Survivial Study Group. Randomised trial of cholesterol lowering in 4444 patients with coronary heart disease: the Scandinavian Simvastatin Survival Study (4S). *Lancet* 1994; **344:** 1383-9.

4. Sacks FM, Pfeffer MA, Moye LA, et al. The effect of pravastatin on coronary events after myocardial infarction in patients with average cholesterol levels. Cholesterol and recurrent events trial investigators. *N Engl J Med* 1996; **335:** 1001-9.

5. The Long-Term Intervention with Pravastatin in Ischaemic Disease (LIPID) Study Group. Prevention of cardiovascular events and death with pravastatin in patients with coronary heart disease and a broad range of initial cholesterol levels. *N Engl J Med* 1998; **339:** 349-57.

6. Wray R, Neil A, Rees A. Hyperlipidaemia in childhood: a screening strategy. UK recommendations. In: Neil A, Rees A, Taylor C, eds. *Hyperlipidaemia in childhood.* London: Royal College of Physicians, 1996; 99-105.

7. Hulley S, Grady D, Bush T, et al. Randomized trial of estrogen plus progestin for secondary prevention of coronary heart disease in postmenopausal women. Heart and Estrogen/progestin Replacement Study (HERS) Research Group. *JAMA* 1998; **280:** 605-13.

8. Wood D, Durrington P, Poulter N, McInnes G, Rees A, Wray R. Joint British recommendations on prevention of coronary heart disease in clinical practice. *Heart* 1998; **80 (Suppl 2):** S1-S29.

9. Standing Medical Advisory Committee. SMAC statement on use of statins. London: Department of Health, 1997 (Executive Letter: EL (97) 41).

10. Wood D, De Backer G, Faergeman O, Graham I, Mancia G, Pyorala K. Prevention of coronary heart disease in clinical practice: recommendations of the Second Joint Task Force of European and other Societies on Coronary Prevention. *Atherosclerosis* 1998; **140:** 199-270.

11. Anderson KM, Odell PM, Wilson PW, Kannel WB. Cardiovascular disease risk profiles. *Am Heart J* 1991; **121:** 293-8.

12. West of Scotland Coronary Prevention Group. Influence of pravastatin and plasma lipids on clinical events in the West of Scotland Coronary Prevention Study (WOSCOPS). *Circulation* 1998; **97:** 1440-5.

13. National Cholesterol Education Program Expert Panel, Summary of the second report of the National Cholesterol Education Program (NECP) Expert Panel on Detection, Evaluation and Treatment of High Blood Cholesterol in Adults (Adult Treatment Panel II). *JAMA* 1993; **269:** 3015-23.

14. Ul Haq I, Ramsay LE, Pickin JN, Yeo WW, Jackson PR, Payne JN. Lipid lowering for prevention of coronary heart disease: what policy now? *Clin Sci (Colch)* 1996; **91:** 773-4.

15. Durrington PN, Prais H, Bhatnagar D, et al. Indications for cholesterol-lowering medication: comparison of risk-assessment methods. *Lancet* 1999; **353:** 278-81.

16. Durrington PN. Triglycerides are more important in atherosclerosis than epidemiology has suggested. *Atherosclerosis* 1998; **141 (Suppl.1)** S57-62.

17. Hokanson JE, Austin MA. Plasma triglyceride level is a risk factor for cardiovascular disease independent of high-density lipoprotein cholesterol: a meta-analysis of population based prospective studies. *J Cardiovasc Risk* 1996; **3:** 213-21.

18. Tang JL, Armitage JM, Lancaster T, Silagy CA, Fowler GH, Neil HAW. Systematic review of dietary intervention trials to lower total cholesterol in free-living subjects. *BMJ* 1998; **316:** 1213-20.

19. Oliver MF. It is more important to increase the intake of unsaturated fats than to decrease the intake of saturated fats: evidence from clinical trials relating to ischemic heart disease. *Am J Clin Nutr* 1997; **66 (suppl):** 980S-986S.

Hypercholesterolaemia: secondary prevention

Alan Rees
Consultant Physician
University Hospital of Wales
Heath Park
Cardiff CF4 4XW

Introduction

Large clinical trials with different 3-hydroxy-3-methylglutaryl[l] coenzyme A (HMG CoA) reductase inhibitors (statins) have demonstrated that lipid-lowering therapy reduces cardiovascular morbidity and mortality, and overall mortality, in both patients with established coronary heart disease (CHD)[1,2] (secondary prevention) and those at high risk of developing CHD[3] (primary prevention). The debate about cholesterol lowering has, therefore, moved from questions of efficacy and safety to those of cost, cost-effectiveness and patient selection.

Which patients to treat

Patients vary enormously in their risk of developing CHD. Individuals with predictors of CHD, such as hypertension, dyslipidaemia, smoking and diabetes mellitus are at high risk relative to the general population, particularly if more than one risk-factor co-exists in the same individual. In general, however, those with clinically overt atherosclerotic disease are at highest risk and are given highest priority in prevention strategies[4]. Thus, the distinction between primary and secondary prevention is somewhat arbitrary, but reflects the reality of clinical practice, as such patients are easily identified, having already presented to the medical services.

The evidence for lifestyle modification and lipid lowering in secondary prevention comes from epidemiology and randomised control trials, which have mostly been undertaken after a myocardial infarction (MI). However, more limited data from patients with unstable angina, or in those who have undergone coronary artery bypass surgery are, in general, concordant with the results obtained in patients post-MI. The Joint British Recommendations for the Prevention of Coronary Heart Disease in Clinical Practice[5] emphasise that individual CHD risk-factors should not be considered in isolation, and that an integrated approach to management should be adopted in the strategy for prevention of CHD in patients with established disease. The following areas are important:

Lifestyle (smoking, diet);
Blood pressure control;
Modification of serum lipids;
Control of diabetes mellitus; and
Cardioprotective drug treatment (aspirin, beta-blockers, angiotensin-converting-enzyme [ACE] inhibitors).

Evidence for benefit of lowering cholesterol

Both increased total serum cholesterol and low concentrations of the high-density lipoprotein (HDL) cholesterol subfraction continue to be risk-factors for recurrent CHD events after MI[4], and evidence that patients with established CHD benefit from cholesterol reduction is exceptionally strong. The most comprehensive meta-analysis conducted before the statin trials (see below) included 21 trials in patients with CHD investigating diet, drugs (clofibrate, gemfibrozil, cholestyramine, colestipol and niacin) or partial ileal bypass surgery[6,7]. The mean serum cholesterol was 6 mmol/L and an average 10% reduction in cholesterol was associated with a 10% reduction in CHD mortality (confidence intervals 3-16%; p = 0.004). Trials using coronary angiography to assess the effects of lipid lowering have also demonstrated slower rates of progression and higher rates of regression, irrespective of the interventions employed. However, concerns have been expressed about the safety of some of the older drugs used[8].

The landmark trials are those using statins as the lipid lowering intervention. These are 4S (Scandinavian Simvastatin Survival Study)[1], CARE (Cholesterol And Recurrent Events)[2] and LIPID (Long-term Intervention with Pravastatin in Ischaemic Heart Disease)[9]. In summary, these trials have demonstrated that reduction of total serum cholesterol and low-density lipoprotein (LDL) cholesterol in the region of $25 - 35\%$ using statins reduced CHD mortality by approximately the same degree. Analysis of pre-specified subgroups of patients showed that the benefit was the same regardless of age, gender or whether the patient had diabetes mellitus. Moreover, patients with unstable angina benefited to the same degree as those post-MI. After integrating the different entry criteria for patients in each of these trials, the consensus interpretation of the data is, simply, that statin therapy should be introduced in all patients with established coronary heart disease, whose serum cholesterol is 5 mmol/L or more.

Some trials have shown that cholesterol lowering, in the context of secondary CHD prevention, reduces the risk of stroke[2,9]. Controlled trials are currently investigating the potential benefit of such therapy in patients with cerebrovascular disease. Similarly, patients with atherosclerosis of the aorta or peripheral vascular disease are at very high risk of co-existent CHD and may also benefit from cholesterol lowering.

When to measure cholesterol
Shortly after MI, concentrations of total, LDL and HDL cholesterol decrease[10]. Other types of physical stress, such as intercurrent illness and surgery, have a similar effect. The reduction in serum cholesterol after MI usually lasts about six weeks, but can be longer if recovery is complicated. In practice, a lipid profile obtained within 24 hours of the onset of symptoms will give a reasonable indication of the lipid profile before the acute event. Patients are well motivated to make lifestyle changes at this stage and discovery of a raised total cholesterol can focus their attention on the need for dietary change and weight loss.

Notwithstanding the lipid profile obtained during the acute phase, it is essential to obtain a further sample after six weeks to determine the need for drug treatment and, for those already on a statin, whether the dose needs to be increased. This also provides an opportunity for a fasting plasma glucose to be measured.

Dietary advice

The dietary recommendations made by the Committee on Medical Aspects of Food (COMA) panel on diet and cardiovascular disease[11], intended for the population as a whole, state that total dietary intake of fats should be reduced to 35% or less of the total energy intake, saturated fat intake to no more than one-third of fat intake, and cholesterol intake to less than 300 mg daily. Early trials of diet in patients with CHD utilising reduced saturated fat intake did not give convincing results. More recent trials, utilising diets low in saturated fat and supplemented with polyunsaturated fatty acids, mainly from omega-3 fatty acids (three helpings of oily fish per week, fish oil capsules and alpha-linoleic acid margarine (eg, 'Flora', 'Vitalite' or own brand sunflower oil based margarines) have shown significant reductions in coronary mortality and improved survival[12,13].

It is unlikely that these benefits are achieved through quantitative modification of the lipid profile since they had minimal effect on it, and patients in these studies were not selected because of hyperlipidaemia. However, more subtle qualitative changes in lipoprotein composition remain a possible mechanism. Thus, in patients with CHD, not only should the general recommendations be reinforced but an increase in the use of monounsaturated and polyunsaturated fats (particularly from omega-3 sources), as well as in fresh fruit and vegetables, should also be emphasised. Although there are no controlled clinical trials of reducing obesity following the development of CHD, it seems sensible to include weight reduction in dietary advice when appropriate, given the known association of obesity with dyslipidaemia, hypertension and type 2 diabetes mellitus.

Management strategy

Dietary advice should be given to all patients. However, only a small proportion of patients will achieve cholesterol concentrations below 5 mmol/L (LDL cholesterol 3 mmol/L or less) with diet alone. Also, the strategy of waiting for the results of the cholesterol concentration at six weeks, before initiating drug treatment, leads to many patients missing effective treatment. The pragmatic approach is to ensure that all patients admitted with unstable angina or acute MI with a random total cholesterol concentration more than 6 mmol/L should, in addition to dietary advice, be prescribed a statin before discharge with a clear statement about the lifelong need for such therapy in the hospital summary.

Patients whose cholesterol concentration at six or more weeks after their acute hospital admission is still 5 mmol/L or more, following dietary advice, should also be given a statin. Those with a cholesterol concentration less than 5 mmol/L should be monitored, at least annually, because despite dietary advice, lipid-lowering therapy may still be needed later. Although long-term survivors of MI were excluded from the intervention studies and are possibly at slightly lower risk, many experts would initiate treatment once their total cholesterol concentrations exceeded 5 mmol/L. Younger patients presenting with MI or unstable angina (men aged less than 55 years and women aged less than 60 years) whose cholesterol is more than 5 mmol/L, or any patient whose serum cholesterol is particularly high (more than 8 mmol/L), may have familial hypercholesterolaemia or another inherited form of dyslipidaemia and their first degree relatives should be invited for screening.

Statins are the preferred drugs for secondary prevention in patients with CHD, as the best evidence of benefit from cholesterol lowering in secondary prevention comes from randomised controlled trials using them. The choice of statin and starting dose represent tensions between cost effectiveness and an evidence-based approach. The controlled trials of secondary prevention used pravastatin (CARE, LIPID) and

216   *Prescribers' Journal 1999 Vol.39 No.4*

simvastatin (4S). It is possible that the benefits of cholesterol lowering in this context may be a class effect of the statins, but differences in tolerability or toxicity cannot be excluded and the results of appropriate outcome studies with other licensed statins are yet to be published. Also, while the trials used either fixed maximum doses or doses titrated from an intermediate level, in practice many patients are started on a low dose with subsequent titration. The effectiveness of this strategy crucially depends on increasing the dose every four to six weeks to achieve the target levels of the intervention trials of total cholesterol less than 5.0 mmol/L or LDL cholesterol less than 3.0 mmol/L. Patients failing to reach this target should be referred to a specialist clinic.

A meta-analysis of clinical trials suggests that fibric acid derivatives also decrease CHD incidence but may increase overall mortality[8]. Any benefit is likely to be more pronounced in combined dyslipidaemia, where both serum cholesterol and triglycerides are raised. Because of the possibility of harm with fibrates, a statin is the initial choice of therapy, even in combined hyperlipidaemia - particularly when the triglycerides are less than 5 mmol/L. In especially high-risk patients with hypertriglyceridaemia persisting despite statin therapy, referral to a specialist lipid clinic is appropriate.

Cost-effectiveness of cholesterol lowering
Recent analyses, based on the results of angiographic regression or outcome studies, have shown that the cost-effectiveness of statin therapy in secondary prevention compares well with some current interventions in cardiovascular disease management[14,15] (see Table 1). Their cost-effectiveness was good in all subgroups studied, under a wide range of clinical and economic conditions.

How well are we doing in the UK?
Despite overwhelming evidence that the management of cardiovascular risk factors in patients with established CHD is beneficial, risk-factor recording and management is substantially sub-optimal and there is considerable potential to improve secondary prevention practice. In

Table 1: *Cost-effectiveness of statins used in secondary prevention compared with other common cardiovascular interventions (costs converted from US dollars)*[16]

Intervention	Cost/QALY
Advice to quit smoking	£800
Beta-blocker post MI	£2200
Statin therapy	£7400

QALY=Quality Adjusted Life Year

ASPIRE[17], a national survey of secondary prevention practice undertaken by the British Cardiac Society shortly after the results of the 4S study were published, 78% of men and 86% of women had a cholesterol reading of 5 mmol/L or more.

Conclusions

- There is good evidence of the benefit of statin therapy post-MI.
- Good clinical practice, based on clinical trial evidence, indicates that target levels post-MI (or in unstable angina) should be a total cholesterol of no more than 5 mmol/L.
- This can be achieved by introducing statin therapy in appropriate doses.
- Treatment with statins is likely to be lifelong and is highly cost-effective.

References

1. Scandinavian Simvastatin Survival Study Group. Randomised trial of cholesterol lowering in 4444 patients with coronary heart disease: the Scandinavian simvastatin survival study (4S). *Lancet* 1994; **344:** 1383-9.
2. Sacks FM, Pfeffer MA, Moyle LA, et al. The effect of pravastatin on coronary events after myocardial infarction in patients with average cholesterol levels. N *Engl J Med* 1996; **335:** 1001-9.
3. Shepherd J, Cobbe SM, Ford I, et. al. Prevention of coronary heart disease with pravastatin in men with hypercholesterolemia. West of Scotland coronary prevention study group. *N Engl J Med* 1995; **333:** 1301-7.

4. Pekkanen J, Linn S, Heiss G, et al. Ten-year mortality from cardiovascular disease in relation to cholesterol level among men with and without pre-existing cardiovascular disease. *N Engl J Med* 1990; **322:** 1700-7.

5. Wood DA, Durrington PN, Poulter N, et al. Joint British recommendations on prevention of coronary heart disease in clinic practice. *Heart* 1998; **80:** Supplement 2 S1-29.

6. Law MR, Wald NJ, Thompson SG. By how much and how quickly does reduction in serum cholesterol concentration lower risk of ischaemic heart disease? *BMJ* 1994; **308:** 367-72.

7. Law MR, Thompson SG, Wald NJ. Assessing possible hazards of reducing serum cholesterol. *BMJ* 1994; **308:** 373-9.

8. Gould AL, Rossouw JE, Santanello NC, Heyse JF, Furberg CD. Cholesterol reduction yields clinical benefit: a new look at old data. *Circulation* 1995; **91:** 2274-82.

9. The Long-term Intervention with Pravastatin in Ischaemic Disease (LIPID) study group. Prevention of cardiovascular events and death with pravastatin in patients with coronary heart disease and a broad range of initial cholesterol levels. *N Engl J Med* 1998; **339:** 1349-57.

10. MBewu AD, Durrington PN, Bulleid S, Mackness MI. The immediate effect of streptokinase on serum lipoprotein(a) concentration and the effect of myocardial infarction on serum lipoprotein(a), apolipoproteins A1 and B, lipids and C-reactive protein. *Atherosclerosis* 1993; **103:** 65-71.

11 Department of Health. *Diet and risk.* Report of the Committee on Medical Aspects of Food Policy (COMA). London: HMSO, 1994.

12. Burr ML, Fehily AM, Gilbert JF. Effects of changes in fat, fish and fibre intakes on death and myocardial reinfarction: diet and reinfarction trial. *Lancet* 1989; **2:** 757-61.

13. de Lorgeril M, Renaud S, Mamelle N, et al. Mediterranean alpha-linolenic acid-rich diet in secondary prevention of coronary heart disease. *Lancet* 1994; **343:** 1454-9.

14. Johanneson M, Jonsson B, Kjekshus J, Olsson AG, Pedersen TR, Wedel H. Cost effectiveness of simvastatin treatment to lower cholesterol levels in patients with coronary heart disease. *N Engl J Med* 1997; **336:** 332-6.

15. Ashraf T, Hay JW, Pitt B, et al. Cost effectiveness of pravastatin in secondary prevention of coronary artery disease. *Am J Cardiol* 1996; **78:** 409-14.

16. Jacobson TA. Improving health outcomes without increasing costs: maximising the full potential of lipid reduction therapy in the primary and secondary prevention of coronary heart disease. *Current Opinion in Lipidology* 1997; **8:** 369-74.

17. Bowker TJ, Clayton TC, Ingham J. A British Cardiac Society survey of potential for the secondary prevention of coronary disease: ASPIRE (Action on Secondary Prevention through Intervention to Reduce Events). *Heart* 1996; **4:** 334-42.

Practical statin prescribing

Indication
- Established coronary heart disease (CHD) (myocardial infarction, angina, ischaemic stroke or peripheral vascular disease) and total cholesterol >5.0 mmol/L.
- Risk of CHD event >3.0% per year (where and when resources permit >1.5% per year) and total cholesterol >5.0 mmol/L.

Important contraindications
- Statins should not be used in pregnancy or breastfeeding.
- Statins should be avoided in active liver disease.

Choice of statin - see articles on pages 202 and 212
- Placebo-controlled evidence of efficacy and safety only for simvastatin and pravastatin.
- Atorvastatin, cerivastatin and fluvastatin may be more cost-effective in terms of cholesterol lowering.

Dosing
- Choice of starting dose may either be based on those used in the trials (simvastatin 20 mg or pravastatin 40 mg) or based on considerations of economy and tolerability, when the lowest dose can be used.
- Whatever starting dose it is essential to titrate upwards (doubling) if total cholesterol > 5.0 mmol/L.

Patient education
- Most statins are most effective when taken in the evening.
- The most important symptomatic adverse effect is myositis. This is rare (<1:10,000) but patients should be asked to report any unexplained muscle pain or weakness. If their creatine phosphokinase >10 x upper limit, attribute to statin and withdraw therapy.

Monitoring

- Only one specimen (pre-treatment) needs to be fasting (can be taken at same time as fasting blood sugar) to detect those with high triglycerides, who should be referred for specialist advice.
- Measure total cholesterol (non-fasting) four to six weeks after starting, or after any dose change.
- Measure liver function tests pre-treatment and at end of dose titration.

Important drug interactions

- Simvastatin may enhance the effect of warfarin.
- Other lipid-lowering drugs, macrolide antibiotics (clarithromycin and erythromycin), and cyclosporin may increase risk of myositis with statins.
- Imidazole antifungal drugs (effects of statins may be enhanced).

Flecainide

S Mark Sopher
Specialist Registrar
David E Ward
Consultant
Cardiology Department
St George's Hospital
London SW17 0QT

Introduction

Flecainide, a fluorinated derivative of the anti-arrhythmic drug procainamide, has anti-arrhythmic properties. However, the demonstration that it can also cause arrhythmias[1], particularly in patients with severe cardiac disease, and those started on high doses, led to a general re-appraisal of its role in anti-arrhythmic therapy, and it is now used for treating atrial fibrillation, and occasionally other arrhythmias, in the absence of structural heart disease.

Mechanism of action

Flecainide falls within class Ic of the Vaughan-Williams classification of anti-arrhythmic drugs[2]: it blocks the fast inward sodium current in cardiac tissue and has little effect on the duration of the action potential. It also reduces automaticity (the tendency for myocardial cells to depolarise spontaneously). These properties give flecainide the potential to treat all forms of tachyarrhythmia, although with the potential also to promote re-entrant arrhythmias.

Pharmacokinetics

Flecainide is well absorbed orally, has a large volume of distribution, and is eliminated both by hepatic metabolism to inactive metabolites, and by renal excretion of unchanged drug. The average half-life is about 14 hours, but the range is wide - from 3-24 hours.

Clinical use

The use of flecainide, like other class I anti-arrhythmic drugs, is generally limited to patients with structurally normal hearts, so all patients should be examined to exclude significant valvular disease or heart failure, and have a 12-lead electrocardiogram to exclude previous myocardial infarction, before treatment is begun. The main use of flecainide now is to terminate symptomatic acute atrial fibrillation (of less than 48 hours' duration), and to prevent the recurrence of atrial fibrillation. Slow intravenous infusion of flecainide will restore sinus rhythm in 70-95% of patients with acute atrial fibrillation[3], which is comparable to other class I anti-arrhythmic drugs.

The dosage is up to 2 mg per kilogram bodyweight, to a total dose of up to 150 mg, given over 10-30 minutes with continuous electrocardiographic monitoring. This can be followed, if necessary, by an infusion of 1.5 mg per kg, given over one hour. If necessary, a further infusion of 100-250 micrograms per kg per hour may be given for up to 24 hours, or up to a total dosage of 600 mg if this is reached first. Once sinus rhythm has been restored, flecainide can be given orally in a dosage of 50 mg twice-daily, increased if required to 100 mg twice-daily.

Flecainide terminates atrial fibrillation in up to 50% of patients with pre-excitation syndromes, eg, Wolff-Parkinson-White syndrome, and reduces the ventricular rate in the remainder[3]. In common with other class I anti-arrhythmic drugs, flecainide has little effect in terminating atrial flutter, and may be dangerous because it can slow the atrial rate sufficiently for the atrioventricular block to change from 2:1 to 1:1, paradoxically causing an increase in ventricular rate fibrillation[4]. It may also make patients with atrial fibrillation more prone to atrial flutter, possibly with haemodynamic deterioration[4].

Orally administered flecainide can be used to maintain sinus rhythm after pharmacological or electrical cardioversion, and is better tolerated than quinidine or disopyramide. It also reduces the frequency and duration of episodes of paroxysmal atrial fibrillation: the overall effect is variable but generally has a clinically useful effect of increasing the duration of sinus rhythm between episodes of atrial fibrillation[5], and probably reduces the ventricular rate if a paroxysm occurs. Again, the dosage is 50 mg twice-daily, increased if necessary to a maximum of 100 mg twice-daily. In this context it may unmask subclinical sinus node disease resulting in sinus bradycardia. Flecainide can also effectively terminate paroxysmal supraventricular tachycardia, but has largely been superseded by adenosine in this indication.

Early clinical studies demonstrated the ability of flecainide to suppress ventricular premature beats by over 80% in over 80% of patients[4] and it is still occasionally a valuable option in the treatment of the small proportion of troublesome ventricular arrhythmias that occur in patients demonstrated to have structurally normal hearts.

Contraindications, adverse effects, and interactions

Flecainide increases the risk of ventricular arrhythmia and sudden death three-fold in asymptomatic patients with ectopic beats after myocardial infarction[1] and should, therefore, not be used in patients with evidence of previous MI. It is also relatively contraindicated in those with heart failure, haemodynamically significant valvular heart disease, or cardiomyopathy.

Flecainide causes dose-dependent widening of the QRS-complex. The potential for ventricular pro-arrhythmia (tachycardia or fibrillation, but very rarely torsade de pointes) also appears to be dose-related, even in those with structurally normal hearts[4].

Hepatic or renal impairment can reduce elimination of flecainide, and cause an increase in plasma concentrations. Therapeutic drug monitoring to maintain plasma concentrations below 1 mg/L may be valuable in these circumstances.

Flecainide can depress myocardial function and cause overt heart failure. The pacing threshold may increase more than twofold[5]. Hepatic damage, peripheral neuropathy, and pulmonary fibrosis have been reported, rarely. Minor adverse effects include blurred vision, dizziness, and nausea.

Significant pharmacokinetic interactions exist with several drugs, including other anti-arrhythmic drugs[4]. Flecainide increases serum digoxin concentration by around 20%; amiodarone significantly increases plasma flecainide concentrations; co-administration with propranolol increases the plasma concentrations of both drugs. Fluoxetine and cimetidine also increase flecainide concentrations. Negatively inotropic drugs, such as propranolol, verapamil, and disopyramide, increase the risk of heart failure with flecainide.

Drugs such as terfenadine, astemizole, tricyclic antidepressants, potassium-losing diuretics, quinine and halofantrine, all of which can prolong the QT interval, increase the risks of serious ventricular arrhythmias.

Conclusions
- Flecainide is useful in the treatment and prophylaxis of atrial fibrillation.
- As flecainide increases the mortality in patients following myocardial infarction, can provoke ventricular arrhythmias, and worsen heart failure, clinical and electrocardiographic assessment to exclude structural heart disease, previous infarction, or heart failure, are essential before using it.
- Flecainide interacts with many other drugs.

References
1. The Cardiac Arrhythmia Suppression Trial (CAST) Investigators. Preliminary report: effect of encainide and flecainide on mortality in a randomized trial of arrhythmia suppression after myocardial infarction. *N Engl J Med* 1989; **321:** 406-12.
2. Vaughan-Williams EM. *Classification of anti-arrhythmic drugs.* In: Sandoc E, Flensted-Jensen E, Oleson ICH, eds. Symposium on cardiac arrhythmias. Sodertaije, Sweden: AB Astra; 1970; 449.

3. Kingma JH, Suttorp MJ. Acute phamacological conversion of atrial fibrillation and flutter: the role of flecainide, propafenone and verapamil. *Am J Cardiol* 1992; **70:** 56A-60A.

4. Falk RH, Fogel RI. Flecainide. *J Cardiovasc Electrophysiol* 1994; **5:** 964-981.

5. Anderson JL, Gilbert EM, Alpert BL, et al. Prevention of symptomatic recurrences of paroxysmal atrial fibrillation in patients initially tolerating antiarrhythmic therapy. A multicenter, double-blind, crossover study of flecainide and placebo with trans telephonic monitoring. Flecainide Supraventricular Tachycardia Study Group. *Circulation* 1989; **82:** 1557-70.

Anorexia nervosa and bulimia nervosa

Janet Treasure
Consultant Psychiatrist
Maudsley Hospital
London SE5 8AZ

Introduction

Bulimia nervosa was first described in 1979, and an exponential rise in the number of cases presenting for treatment followed. The risk of developing bulimia nervosa has risen in each ten-year cohort of women born after the 1950s[1]. In contrast, the balance of evidence is that there has been no recent increase in the number of new cases of anorexia nervosa[2], although the mortality associated with it (which, at 20%, is the highest associated for any psychiatric illness) may be increasing[3]. This deteriorating course means that prevalence of anorexia nervosa has also increased. The lifetime risk among women of developing bulimia nervosa is now 8% while that of anorexia nervosa is 3%. For both disorders the risk among men is approximately ten-fold lower.

Diagnosis and recognition

Anorexia nervosa is a condition of weight loss, with a body-mass index (BMI) below 17.5, caused by food avoidance secondary to psychosocial conflict. The diagnosis of anorexia nervosa is usually not a problem for the clinician. Apart from weight loss the obvious physical features are poor peripheral circulation, low blood pressure, bradycardia and the development of lanugo hair. Patients with anorexia nervosa perceive themselves to be fat and wish to be thin. To achieve this they indulge in rituals and compulsions to control their eating, and undertake excess physical activity. They can be hostile and irritable. A history from an informant will clarify whether there appears to be a planned strategy to produce weight loss, either by calorie restriction or by the use of laxatives, vomiting or over-exercise. However, the patient will either be reluctant to accept the diagnosis or to collaborate with any form of treatment.

Bulimia nervosa, in contrast, is a condition of over-eating associated with the use of laxatives, vomiting, or over-exercise to control weight. The eating behaviour of patients with bulimia nervosa fluctuates from fasting to binges, despite preoccupation with body weight and shape. Such patients have low self-esteem and may become depressed. Often ashamed about their problem, they may not ask for help directly but rather allude to the subject of diets or vomiting in a consultation for other things.

The cognitive component of the mental state in both disorders is coloured by culture and is not always present in the same form. The overvalued idea(s) underlying the behaviour may be covert or confused.

Investigations
Investigations are of little help in confirming the diagnosis and should be limited to those necessary to exclude other likely diagnoses or important consequences of starvation and other weight control measures. Important alternative illnesses to consider in patients with weight loss are inflammatory bowel disease, infection - especially tuberculosis and HIV- endocrinological disorders such as hypopituitarism, diabetes and Addison's disease, and malignant disease. A minimal set of investigations might include a full blood count and erythrocyte sedimentation rate, urea and electrolytes, and liver function tests. In patients with an atypical presentation, further investigations such as computerised tomography brain scan might be considered to exclude an intracerebral malignancy. Anorexia and bulimia alone may be associated with minor laboratory abnormalities - typically low haemoglobin, white cell count and urea. Other electrolyte disturbances eg, low sodium and potassium and high bicarbonate - due to loss of acidic gastric contents - may be seen in patient with frequent vomiting.

One important complication of anorexia is a reduced bone mass and patients whose duration of disease exceeds one year should have a scan for bone density.

Management
Anorexia nervosa
The most difficult part of management is for clinician and patient to agree a common goal for change. People with anorexia nervosa are, at best, ambivalent about help to change and, at worst, totally resistant. Because of this it may be useful to use the technique of motivational interviewing[4]. It is usually helpful to involve parents in treatment but the form and intensity of this will depend on the age and maturity of the patient. Specific education about the disorder and about interpersonal functioning is often given. Two books have been written for the family and individual but their use has not been evaluated[5,6]. Similarly, although there is a wide network of self-help groups, their efficacy has not been investigated.

Vitamin supplements are not generally advised and most effort should be expended in encouraging food intake. The disease should be monitored by regular weighing and patients with a BMI below 17 for longer than three months despite simple measures should be referred to a psychiatrist with a specific interest in eating disorders. Admission should be requested for patients where the BMI is less than 13.

Anorexia nervosa is one of the conditions for which patients can be formally admitted under the Mental Health Act. However it is crucially important that they are admitted to a unit which specialises in eating disorders. In such units force-feeding should rarely, if ever, be necessary. Although inpatient treatment is effective in the short term, relapse is common and a pattern of repeated admissions may develop. Several centres within the UK have found that many patients can be managed with specialised outpatient psychotherapy. Others have recently developed day-patient services. The long-term effectiveness of any of these models of service is unknown.

Essential facets of treatment are to:

Find out what are the patient's beliefs about their illness;

Develop a good therapeutic alliance;

Explore the links between behaviour and underlying beliefs about self; *and*

Match therapeutic processes to readiness to change.

Medication

There is no evidence that medication can improve upon the weight gain that can be achieved by inpatient care given by a skilled nursing team. However, the place of medication in other forms of service has not been evaluated. For example, early reports of a randomised study suggest that fluoxetine may prevent relapse once patients have reached target weight in hospital. However, in other areas specific serotonin reuptake inhibitors (SSRIs) have been shown to be less effective in low oestrogen states and their routine use in patients with anorexia noervosa cannot be recommended without further studies. Poor gastric emptying is a feature of anorexia nervosa and may lead to feelings of fullness and lack of hunger. Cisapride reduced such symptoms more than placebo[7] but did not increase weight gain. A minority of women with anorexia nervosa have a prolonged QT interval, which is associated with sudden death. Cisapride should therefore be reserved for patients with severe symptoms and then only used after an electrocardiographic examination has excluded prolongation of the QT interval.

Osteoporosis develops in anorexia nervosa because of low bone turnover, with formation falling behind resorption. One randomised study of hormone replacement therapy (HRT)[8] did not find it to be effective in increasing bone density. However a post-hoc analysis of the subgroup that continued to lose weight suggested that HRT may prevent further bone loss in persistent anorexia nervosa.

Bulimia nervosa

Effective management of bulimia nervosa is much more clearly defined than for anorexia nervosa. The first development was the establishment of specific forms of psychotherapy, including cognitive behaviour therapy. These were found to be effective in relieving symptoms in over one-half of the cases[9]. Much of the didactic content of these forms of therapy was then written into manuals for the sufferer to use[9,10]. People with binge eating disorders without intense weight control measures can obtain a significant improvement using such manuals alone[11], whereas in bulimia nervosa some additional form of therapeutic guidance produces significantly better results[12].

Essential facets of treatment are:
Evaluate the level of motivation for all symptoms (patients will want to give up bingeing but will be more reluctant to give up weight control);
Address ambivalence;
Educate about nutrition and the control of appetite;
Monitor behaviour and thoughts with a diary; *and*
Connect symptoms with beliefs about self.

Medication
Several classes of antidepressant drugs, including the tricyclics and SSRIs, have been more effective than placebo in the short-term treatment of bulimia nervosa. In the two largest studies published so far, fluoxetine at doses (60 mg daily) above those usually used in the treatment of depression has been shown to be effective in reducing bulimic and depressive symptoms in bulimia nervosa patients. The remission rate was reported to be about 25% at the end of the eight weeks trial[13] and merely 18% at the end of the 16 week trial[14]. The performance of drugs is believed to be inferior to that of psychotherapy, which produces more substantial and long-lasting change. However, there is some evidence that antidepressants may be useful supplements to psychotherapy[15] and may have a place with the more minimal interventions such as guided self-care.

Conclusions
- The prevalence and severity of anorexia nervosa may be increasing.
- Both the incidence and prevalence of bulimia nervosa is increasing.

- There is little evidence on which to base the management of anorexia nervosa, and primary care clinicians should limit themselves to education and encouragement. When weight loss persists, referral to a psychiatrist with a special interest should be considered.
- The most effective form of psychotherapy for bulimia nervosa is cognitive behavioural therapy. Such an approach can be successfully distilled into forms of self-care.

References

1. Kendler KS, McLean C, Neale M, et al. The genetic epidemiology of bulimia nervosa. *Am J Psych* 1991; **148:** 1627-37.
2. Fombonne E. Anorexia nervosa. No evidence of an increase. *Br J Psych* 1995; **166:** 462-71.
3. Moller-Madsen S, Nystrup J, Nielsen S. Mortality of anorexia nervosa in Denmark during the period 1970-1987. *Acta Psychiatr Scand* 1996; **94:** 454-9.
4. Miller WR, Rollnick S. *Motivational Interviewing: Preparing People to Change Addictive Behaviour.* New York: Guildford Press, 1991.
5. Crisp AH, Joughin N, Halek C, Bowyer C. *Anorexia nervosa. The wish to change.* Hove: Psychology Press, 1991.
6. Treasure J. *Anorexia nervosa: a survival guide for families, friends and sufferers.* Hove: Psychology Press, 1987.
7. Szmukler GI, Young GP, Miller G, Lichtenstein M, Binns DS. A controlled trial of cisapride in anorexia nervosa. *Int J Eating Disord* 1995; **17:** 345-57.
8. Klibanski A, Biller BM, Schoenfeld DA, Herzog DB, Saxe VC. The effects of estrogen administration on trabecular bone loss in young women with anorexia nervosa. *J Clin Endocrinol Metab* 1995; **80:** 898-904.
9. Fairburn CG. Overcoming Binge Eating. New York: Guildford, 1995.
10. Schmidt U, Treasure J. *Getting Better Bit(e) by Bit(e). Survival kit for sufferers of bulimia nervosa and binge eating disorders.* Lawrence Erlbaum, 1993.
11. Carter JC, Fairburn CG. Cognitive behavioural self help for binge eating disorder: a controlled effectiveness study. *J Consult Clin Psychol* 1998; **66:** 616-23.
12. Thiels C, Schmidt U, Treasure J, Garthe R, Troop N. Guided self change for bulimia nervosa incorporating a self-care manual. *Am J Psych* 1998; **155:** 947-53.
13. Fluoxetine Bulimia Nervosa Collaborative Study Group. Fluoxetine in the treatment of bulimia nervosa. A multicenter, placebo-controlled, double-blind trial. *Arch Gen Psychiatry* 1992; **49:** 139-47.

14. Goldstein DJ, Wilson MG, Thompson VL, Potvin JH, Rampey AH Jr. Long-term fluoxetine treatment of bulimia nervosa. Fluoxetine Bulimia Nervosa Research Group. *Br J Psychiatry* 1995; **166**: 660-6.
15. Walsh BT, Wilson GT, Loeb KL, et al. Medication and psychotherapy in the treatment of bulimia nervosa. *Am J Psychiatry* 1997; **154**: 523-31.

Hypercalcaemia

David Heath
Consultant Physician
Selly Oak Hospital
Birmingham B29 6JD

Introduction

The upper limit of normal of the serum calcium concentration in most laboratories is 2.60 mmol/L, if associated with normal serum protein concentrations. In this situation, total calcium concentration is a good predictor of ionised calcium. In malignancy, where serum albumin is frequently reduced, the total calcium concentration may underestimate the ionised calcium concentration. This can be overcome, to a degree, by a 'protein-corrected' calcium concentration*. The prevalence of hypercalcaemia varies considerably with the population studied. Prevalence rates of primary hyperparathyroidism are usually quoted as being 1 in 1,000. It is rare in young, healthy adults, increases considerably after the age of 50 years, and is three times more common in women.

In malignancy, the prevalence varies considerably between individual tumours: it is very rare in colonic cancer but common in breast cancer, myeloma and most tumours of squamous cell origin. Overall, around 10% of malignancies may be associated with hypercalcaemia at some stage of their natural history.

---

*measured total calcium concentration (mmol/L) + (40- serum albumin concentration in grams/L)/40

Aetiology and pathogenesis

The causes of hypercalcaemia, with an indication of their frequency of occurrence, are shown in Table 1. The cause can usually be readily identified from the mode of presentation and a careful history.

Table 1: *Causes of hypercalcaemia*

Common
Primary hyperparathyroidism
Malignancy
Chronic renal failure due to complicating hyperparathyroidism and
 treatment with calcium and vitamin D metabolites

Uncommon
Familial benign hypercalcaemia
Sarcoidosis
Vitamin D therapy (outside renal failure)
Milk-alkali syndrome
Thyrotoxicosis

Rare
Various causes beyond the scope of this article: see reference 6.

Primary hyperparathyroidism, today, is typically a mild or asymptomatic disease often brought to light by routine investigations, and it is unusual for patients to be or to appear unwell. In contrast, the hypercalcaemia of malignancy is usually associated with a much more serious clinical state because it usually complicates existing, advanced malignancy not responding to treatment. It is exceptional for hypercalcaemia to be the first sign of an occult malignancy[1]. Patients are therefore unwell, deteriorating as the hypercalcaemia develops, which may happen rapidly over days or weeks, increasing the likelihood of symptoms. It is caused by humoral agents produced by the tumour, in particular by parathyroid hormone-related peptide (PTHrP) which acts on the PTH receptor but is not detected by modern two-site PTH assays[2]. Bone secondaries per se are rarely a cause of hypercalcaemia, and there is no correlation between hypercalcaemia and the extent of skeletal involvement.

Hypercalcaemia due to malignancy is often identified before it causes severe symptoms and clinicians should be aware that, in patients with malignancy, hypercalcaemia may occur. Routine monitoring of serum calcium concentration is important in patients with clinical disease, and at any time that symptoms worsen. Malaise, nausea and constipation can so easily be attributed to the malignancy or to the adverse effects of treatment. Unless effective treatment of the malignancy is possible, the hypercalcaemia is unlikely to resolve and will usually worsen.

Familial benign hypercalcaemia (FBH), also known as familial hypocalciuric hypercalcaemia, is being recognised more frequently, but can very readily be confused with asymptomatic primary hyperparathyroidism. FBH is an inherited condition in which there is an abnormality of the calcium-sensing receptor which enables the parathyroid and renal tubular cells to recognise the ambient ionised calcium concentration. As a consequence, serum calcium concentrations are slightly to moderately raised throughout patients' lives. Typically, this is associated with normal PTH concentrations and there are no symptoms[3]. Apart from the very rare occurrence of severe hypercalcaemia in affected neonates, individuals do not suffer any adverse consequences of the disorder.

A drug history should elicit treatment with vitamin D but can easily miss treatment with proprietary indigestion preparations high in bicarbonates, eg, 'Rennies', which can cause the milk-alkali syndrome.

Investigation and clinical features

Hypercalcaemia may present as follows:

Chance discovery of hypercalcaemia during the investigation of an unconnected condition

This is now the commonest mode of presentation of primary hyperparathyroidism. About one-half of patients are asymptomatic, whilst most of the remainder have mild, non-specific symptoms such as tiredness, lethargy, and mild aches and pains. The demonstration of a raised or high normal serum PTH concentration measured by a specific assay confirms the diagnosis. Further diagnostic investigation is usually not indicated, but caution should be shown in asymptomatic patients whose serum PTH is not clearly raised. Here, the main differential diagnosis is FBH, in which serum PTH concentration is usually well within the normal range, although occasionally it may be high. Although in FBH the serum magnesium concentration tends to be towards the high side of normal and the urine calcium excretion low, values overlap extensively with those values seen in primary hyperparathyroidism. The best way of supporting the diagnosis of FBH is to demonstrate a hypercalcaemic parent, sibling or child.

Patient presents with symptoms

The patient presents with symptoms of more severe hypercalcaemia (nausea, vomiting, polydipsia, polyuria, constipation) or of underlying disease, usually malignancy. Where malignancy is known to be present, serum PTH, if measured, would be low. If there is no clinical evidence of malignancy, the possibility of the rarer, more severe, forms of hyperparathyroidism or some of the less common causes of hypercalcaemia need to be considered and serum PTH level should be measured at an early stage. In hyperparathyroidism it will be clearly raised but in all other conditions it will be lowered. Where malignancy is the cause but not obvious, this is often a low-grade haematological or lymphoid tumour.

Management

An initial decision should be taken on the appropriateness of treating acute severe hypercalcaemia, taking into account the patient's premorbid state, the likelihood of effective management of any co-existing malignancy and the patient's life expectancy. Usually, treatment will be deemed necessary and it has been shown to improve the quality of life of patients with known malignancy. Very occasionally, the patient will be so ill from the malignancy that further treatment is considered inadvisable. If treatment is considered appropriate, an intravenous drip should be started and 3-4 litres of fluid given daily. This will be predominantly sodium chloride 0.9% solution with potassium supplements, as indicated by serum monitoring. Diuretics should only be given when needed to prevent heart failure. Although patients improve with fluid therapy alone, this will never adequately control the hypercalcaemia. For this reason, drug treatment should be started at an early stage in order to obtain gradual control.

Drug treatment of tumour-induced hypercalcaemia
Bisphosphonates
Two bisphosphonates, disodium pamidronate and sodium clodronate, are licensed for this indication; both are effective and vary only in the dosage and frequency of administration. Ideally, a hospital should be familiar with just one regimen. Disodium pamidronate is given as a single infusion of 30-90 mg intravenously over two to four hours (according to serum calcium concentration), or 30 mg daily for three days. Sodium clodronate is given as a single infusion of 1.5 g intravenously over four hours, or 300 mg daily until calcium is controlled (maximum seven days).

Serum calcium concentration falls progressively over several days, usually reaching a nadir after three to five days. This gradual fall produces a marked clinical response. Serious side-effects are uncommon. Fever, 'flu-like symptoms and increased bone pain are most commonly seen with sodium pamidronate. The rare reporting of somnolence and dizziness has led to the advice that outpatients, experiencing these side-effects, should not drive or operate potentially dangerous machinery until symptoms have settled. The commonest adverse effect of sodium clodronate is mild gastrointestinal disturbance.

Intravenous phosphate and ethylenediaminetetraacetic acid (EDTA) have been used in the past and caused a rapid fall, over several hours, in the serum calcium concentration. This was associated with reports of sudden death and such treatments should only be considered where all other forms of management have failed.

Hypercalcaemia is very likely to recur within several weeks, unless the underlying condition, usually cancer, can be treated effectively. If this is not possible, once the hypercalcaemia has been controlled, the addition of oral clodronate 1.6 g daily, increasing, if necessary, to 3.2 g daily, may prevent the recurrence of hypercalcaemia. The dose should be reduced in patients with renal failure, and it is contraindicated in moderate to severe renal failure. With the oral drug, no food or calcium-containing products should be taken at least one hour before or afterwards. If such therapy is ineffective, intermittent infusions of intravenous pamidronate or clodronate can be given every three to four weeks on a day-case basis.

Alternative drugs
High dose oral corticosteroids are almost always ineffective in treating hypercalcaemia associated with solid tumours and only work in hypercalcaemia due to haematological malignancies, vitamin D poisoning and sarcoidosis[4]. In all these situations, bisphosphonates are also effective. Oral corticosteroids, at the lowest effective dose, can be expected to control the hypercalcaemia of sarcoidosis and of many haematological malignancies.

Intravenous or subcutaneous calcitonin is of limited value[5]. It causes a slightly more rapid early fall in calcium concentration than bisphosphonates but there is often a rise in calcium concentration later. It often causes nausea and its use on its own or in combination with other agents is hard to justify.

Drug treatment of hyperparathyroidism
Symptomatic patients are best treated by surgery. There is no evidence that oral bisphosphonates are of value in asymptomatic cases.

Surgical treatment

Surgery rarely helps in the management of hypercalcaemia of malignancy as the disease is usually advanced and disseminated. De-bulking of the tumour mass might be considered in very slow-growing tumours, eg, carcinoids, islet cell tumours and phaeochromocytomas.

Surgery is the most effective treatment of primary hyperparathyroidism, and it is now well accepted that it should only be performed by experienced parathyroid surgeons, with the best results obtained when at least 20 parathyroidectomies are performed per year. The decision whether to operate or to perform pre-operative localisation is best left to a specialist team.

General measures

Patients with hypercalcaemia develop polyuria because the renal tubules become resistant to the action of antidiuretic hormone. This, in return, leads to compensatory polydipsia. As any intercurrent illness can lead to a reduced fluid intake, dehydration, and worsening of the hypercalcaemia, patients should be encouraged to maintain adequate fluid intakes at all times, although it is unrealistic to expect them to maintain intakes of a litre or more above normal. The serum calcium concentration should always be measured if a patient's symptoms alter significantly.

In both the acute and stable situations, instituting a low calcium diet is unnecessary and ineffective. Agents such as cellulose phosphate which block calcium gut absorption are also of no value.

When to treat and when to refer

Acute hypercalcaemia associated with malignancy is best treated in hospital, by an approved protocol which can be audited. Once the hypercalcaemia has been controlled, referral to an oncologist is advisable.

Non-malignant causes of hypercalcaemia rarely need emergency treatment and hyperparathyroidism remains the commonest cause of these other cases. Many cases of asymptomatic hyperparathyroidism or cases with mild symptoms in patients aged over 60 years are managed conservatively. Parathyroid surgery is now recognised to be a specialised procedure that is becoming increasingly restricted to selected centres. Cases that might need surgery are best referred to these centres at an early stage, as this often avoids unnecessary investigations (eg, parathyroid localisation) and treatment (eg, bisphosphonate therapy).

Conclusions

- Hypercalcaemia is a common metabolic abnormality.
- Malignancy and hyperparathyroidism are the two common causes.
- Controlling the hypercalcaemia of malignancy usually improves quality of life; it occasionally requires emergency treatment with intravenous fluids and a bisphosphonate.
- Hyperparathyroidism, when requiring treatment, is best treated surgically by specialist teams.

References

1. Fisken RA, Heath DA, Bold AM. Hypercalcaemia - a hospital survey. *Q J Med* 1980; **49:** 405-18.
2. Grill V, Ho P, Body JJ, et al. Parathyroid hormone-related protein: elevated levels both in humoral hypercalcemia of malignancy and in hypercalcemia complicating metastatic breast cancer. *J Clin Endocrinol Metab* 1991; **73:** 1309-15.
3. Pearce SH. Calcium homeostasis and disorders of the calcium-sensing receptor. *J Roy Coll Physicians Lond* 1998; **32:** 10-4.
4. Percival RC, Yates AJ, Gray RE, Neal FE, Forrest AR, Kanis JA. Role of glucocorticoids in management of malignant hypercalcaemia. *BMJ* 1984; **289:** 287.
5. Heath DA. Treatment of hypercalcaemia of malignancy. *Baillieres Clin Endocrinol Metab* 1990; **4:** 139-45.
6. Bushinsky DA, Monk RD. Calcium. *Lancet* 1998; **352:** 306-11.

Venlafaxine

David S Baldwin
Senior Lecturer in Psychiatry
Mental Health Group
Faculty of Medicine, Health and Biological Sciences
University of Southampton SO14 0YG

Introduction

Venlafaxine is an antidepressant drug belonging to the serotonin/noradrenaline reuptake inhibitor (SNRI) class. It inhibits the presynaptic reuptake of serotonin, of noradrenaline and, to a much lesser extent, dopamine. Serotonin reuptake is inhibited at both low and high doses of venlafaxine; noradrenaline reuptake becomes more prominent with higher doses of the drug[1]. Unlike tricyclic antidepressants (TCAs), it has no affinity for adrenergic, cholinergic or histaminic receptors[1]. It is effective in depressed psychiatric inpatients and outpatients and depressed patients in primary care[2]; it has also been found effective in generalised anxiety disorder (GAD) and may be efficacious in other anxiety disorders and the treatment of certain forms of pain[3]. At present, its licensed indication is for the treatment of depressive illness. When compared with many of the older tricyclic antidepressants, it appears to be well tolerated, and relatively safe in overdose[4].

Clinical pharmacology

Venlafaxine is a bicyclic phenylethylamine compound, with three identified metabolites; the major one, O-desmethyl venlafaxine (ODV) is also pharmacologically active. Peak serum concentrations of venlafaxine are seen within two hours of oral administration; concentrations of ODV rise and decline more slowly, the half-lives being three to four hours for venlafaxine and 10 hours for ODV. The rate of absorption of venlafaxine is not affected by food; it shows less than 30% plasma protein binding; and elimination occurs mainly as ODV and the other metabolites, only 5% of unchanged venlafaxine being recoverable from urine. The pharmacokinetic profile of venlafaxine in elderly subjects is no different to that in those aged under 65 years, but lower doses of the drug are recommended in patients with hepatic or renal insufficiency[5]. Because of the short half-life of venlafaxine, and of ODV, it is advisable to taper dosage on stopping treatment, to minimise discontinuation symptoms.

Mechanism of action
Inhibition of the re-uptake of serotonin and noradrenaline by venlafaxine probably accounts for its activity in behavioural and neurophysiological animal models sensitive to antidepressant drugs, and presumably also accounts for its antidepressant properties in man.

Indications
Venlafaxine has been shown to be antidepressant in double-blind controlled investigations, some of which involved comparison with reference antidepressants[6]. In both its standard release and modified release formulations, venlafaxine has been found superior to placebo, in short- and long-term treatment. In one study, both formulations of venlafaxine showed superiority over placebo: this investigation also found the modified release formulation to be superior to the standard release version, in terms of rating scale response rates after twelve weeks of treatment[7]. The reason for this difference is unclear, and is in need of replication. In comparator studies, venlafaxine has been found at least as effective as, and occasionally superior to, other antidepressant drugs, including imipramine, clomipramine, trazodone and fluoxetine[6]. Studies of higher doses of venlafaxine suggest it may have an earlier onset of action than comparators, but at the expense of a greater risk of adverse effects[4].

Venlafaxine is effective across the range of severity of depression, and has also been found efficacious in chronic or refractory depressive episodes[6,8]. It is probably as effective in elderly patients as in those aged under 65 years[9]. In one study in children and adolescents with major depression there were no differences between venlafaxine and placebo[10]. Efficacy is not reduced in the melancholic sub-type of depression, nor by greater degrees of psychomotor retardation, agitation or anxiety: it has been suggested that the broad utility of venlafaxine in treating depression may be at least partly related to the flexibility in dosage which is possible with the drug[6].

At first, venlafaxine should be prescribed at a dosage of 37.5 mg twice daily. If necessary, the dose should be increased to 75 mg twice daily. In severely depressed or hospitalised patients, the starting dose can be 75 mg twice daily, this being increased if the patient does not show signs of early response, by 75 mg every two to three days to a maximum daily dose of 375 mg. When the clinical situation situation allows, this maximum dosage should then be reduced gradually.

Like the selective SSRIs, and some other antidepressants, venlafaxine may be effective in the treatment of a range of anxiety disorders. In double-blind, placebo-controlled studies it has been found effective in panic disorder, obsessive-compulsive disorder and generalised anxiety disorder (GAD)[3,11]. A recent investigation found that modified-release venlafaxine was superior to placebo, while buspirone was not, in the short term treatment of GAD[12]. However the potential efficacy in the treatment of anxiety disorders requires some confirmation, in particular through the results of longer-term studies[3]. More research is required to see whether the reported analgesic properties of venlafaxine, described in case series of patients with headache, peripheral neuropathic pain or fibromyalgia are confirmed by more rigorous investigations[3].

Adverse effects
Venlafaxine appears to be as well tolerated, or better tolerated than clomipramine, dothiepin, imipramine, maprotiline and trazodone[4]. Nausea occurs in about one-third of patients, especially in the early

stages of treatment, and dizziness, somnolence, dry mouth and insomnia are relatively common[13]. About 20% of patients withdrew from venlafaxine treatment within the first six weeks, citing adverse events as a reason (compared to 6% of placebo-treated patients); after six weeks only 6% of venlafaxine-treated patients withdrew for this reason, compared with 2% of placebo-treated patients. The same trial database shows that the most common adverse effects occur with similar frequency in those aged over or under 65 years[13].

A rise in blood pressure was seen in clinical trials in patients treated with venlafaxine, most often at doses above 200mg per day. The probability of clinically significant increases in blood pressure greater than 15 mmHg, to a diastolic pressure greater than 105 mmHg, increases with dose, being 13% at the highest doses (ie, more than 300 mg per day)[13].

From a total of 1,164 reports of adverse reaction made to the UK Committee on Safety of Medicines up to mid-1997, three cases of thrombocytopenia where described; two of these cases proved fatal, but it is difficult to ascribe causality with any certainty[4]. Although venlafaxine is less likely to cause interference with everyday tasks than older tricyclic antidepressants, performance of skilled tasks (such as driving) may be affected in some patients.

Toxicity and drug-drug interactions

The pooled clinical trial database of 3,082 patients treated with venlafaxine includes 14 patients who took an overdose of the drug. All survived and recovered without sequelae. One patient who ingested 2.75 grams suffered two generalised epileptiform convulsions and a prolongation of the QT interval to 500 milliseconds[13].

Venlafaxine and ODV have only a modest inhibitory effect on the cytochrome P450 system enzymes when compared with some SSRIs, and the potential for drug-drug interactions appears low[14]. Co-administration of venlafaxine with ethanol does not alter the disposition of venlafaxine or ODV. Traditional monoamine oxidase inhibitors (MAOIs) are contra-indicated with venlafaxine, and a 14-day wash-out period is advised between stopping an MAOI and starting venlafaxine. Inadvertent consumption of this combination can lead to the 'serotonin syndrome', consisting of agitation, confusion, myoclonus, hyperreflexia, sweating, shivering, tremor, diarrhoea, inco-ordination and fever[4].

During clinical trials, withdrawal effects from venlafaxine were reported with abrupt discontinuation after daily doses of 150 mg or more ; most discontinuation phenomena occurred within two days of a significant reduction in dosage, and usually resolved within seven days of stopping treatment[15]. In a retrospective survey of 1,060 patients, the most common events after discontinuing treatment, either by tapering or abrupt discontinuation, were headache, reported by 20% of patients (compared with 8% who had received placebo); nausea (venlafaxine, 19% ; placebo, 3%) and dizziness (15% v 2%)[4].

Venlafaxine is contraindicated in patients with known severe hepatic or renal impairment and during pregnancy and breast feeding, when alternative antidepressants should be used. A prescription-event monitoring study showed that 67 pregnancies occurred amongst a total of 8,214 women treated with venlafaxine[4]. When venlafaxine had been given during the first trimester of pregnancy (to 38 patients) there were 25 live births, 7 spontaneous abortions and 6 terminations of pregnancy. More evidence will be needed before any conclusions about the effects of venlafaxine upon the outcome of pregnancy can be made.

Conclusions
- Venlafaxine is an effective antidepressant drug.
- At lower doses it is generally well tolerated; higher doses should be reserved for more severely depressed patients and those with chronic depression who have failed to respond to other treatment.
- More data are required to evaluate its efficacy in anxiety disorder, its toxicity in overdose and safety in pregnancy.

References

1. Horst WD, Preskorn SH. The pharmacology and mode of action of venlafaxine. *Rev Contemp Pharmacother* 1998; **9:** 293-302.

2. Feighner JP. The role of venlafaxine in rational antidepressant therapy. *J Clin Psychiatry* 1994; **55 (suppl A):** 62-8.

3. Nutt D, Johnson FN. Potential applications of venlafaxine. *Rev Contemp Pharmacother* 1998; **9:** 321-31.

4. Sinclair J, Birtwistle J, Baldwin D. The tolerability of venlafaxine. *Rev in Contemp Pharmacother* 1998; **9:** 333-44.

5. Troy SM, Schultz RW, Parker VD, Chiang ST, Blum RA. The effect of renal disease on the disposition of venlafaxine. *Clin Pharnacol Ther* 1994; **56:** 14-21.

6. Burnett FE, Dinan TG. The clinical efficacy of venlafaxine in the treatment of depression. *Rev Contemp Pharmacother* 1998; **9:** 303-20.

7. Derivan AT, Aguiar L, for the Venlafaxine XR 208 Study Group. A double-blind placebo-controlled comparison of venlafaxine and once-daily venlafaxine in patients with major depression. Presented at the World Congress of Biological Psychiatry, Nice, 23-26 June 1997.

8. Nierenberg AA, Feighner JP, Rudolph R, Cole, JA, Sullivan J. Venlafaxine for treatment-resistant unipolar depression. *J Clin Psychopharmacol* 1994; **14:** 419-23.

9. Entsuah AR, Rudolph RL, Chitra R. Effectiveness of venlafaxine treatment in a broad spectrum of depressed patients: a meta-analysis. Psychopharmacol Bull 1995; **31:** 759-766.

10. Mandoki MW, Tapia MR, Tapia MA, Sumner GS, Parker JL. Venlafaxine in the treatment of children and adolescents with major depression. *Psychopharmacol Bull* 1997; **33:** 149-54.

11. Haskins T, Rudolph R, Dallay A, Derivan A, for the Venlafaxine XR 210 Study Group. Double-blind, placebo-controlled study of once-daily venlafaxine XR in outpatients with generalised anxiety disorder. *Eur Neuropsychopharmacol* 1998; **8:** S26.

12. Derivan A, Entsuah R, Haskins T, Rudoph R for the venlafaxine XR 214 Study Group. Double-blind pacebo-comparator controlled study of once-daily venlafaxine XR and buspirone in outpatients with generalised anxiety disorder. *Eur Psychopharmacol* 1998; **8:** S26.

13. Rudolph RL, Derivan AT. The safety and tolerability of venlafaxine hydrochloride: analysis of the clinical trials database. *J Clin Psychopharmacol* 1996; **16 (suppl 2):** 54S-59S.

14. Ereshefsky L. Drug-drug interactions involving antidepressants: focus on venlafaxine. *J Clin Psychophamacol* 1996; **16 (suppl 3):** 37S-50S.

15. Dallal A, Chouinard G. Withdrawal and rebound symptoms associated with abrupt discontinuation of venlafaxine. *J Clin Psychopharmacol* 1998; **18:** 343-4.

Interactions with over-the-counter medicines

Alain Li Wan Po
Professor
Centre for Evidence-Based Pharmacotherapy
Aston University
Birmingham B4 7ET

Introduction

Modern drugs are generally safe, reasonably effective, and of good quality, as stipulated by the Medicines Act 1968. Most medicines, however, have been available only on prescription (prescription-only medicine, POM); some have been available from pharmacies (P), and a small number are on general sale (general sales list, GSL). As no prescription is required for them, P and GSL preparations are referred to as 'over-the-counter' (OTC) medicines. Some preparations, such as H_2-antagonist antacids, are available over-the-counter only in smaller doses and smaller quantities than the equivalent POM preparation.

Over recent years, there has been a trend towards reclassifying prescription-only medicines as P or GSL. This allows easier access to medicines, while users meet some of the costs of treating minor ailments. When deciding whether to reclassify a POM medicine to make it available OTC, drug regulatory authorities consider whether the benefits are sufficient to outweigh the risks. Among the risks that all OTC medicines pose are those of interaction with prescribed medicines, or unwitting overdosage when a branded OTC medicine contains the same active drug as a prescribed medicine. Sometimes, potentially serious adverse effects or drug interactions only become apparent when drugs become available OTC and are used more widely[1]. A recent example is provided by terfenadine, which was made available OTC in 1983, before it was known that some enzyme inhibitors, such as grapefruit juice[2] and the azole antifungal drugs, can inhibit its metabolism, increase the serum terfenadine concentration, and lead to serious cardiac arrhythmia. As a result, the drug is no longer available OTC.

The danger of drug interactions is particularly great for a small group of prescription drugs which have narrow therapeutic ranges. Warfarin is by far the most important, but anti-rejection therapy after transplantation, anticonvulsant drugs, lithium, theophylline (or aminophylline) and many other less commonly used agents fall into the same category. Table 1 sets out some potentially serious drug interactions between OTC and prescribed medicines.

Mechanisms of drug interactions

The mechanisms underlying the common types of drug interaction include:

Enzyme induction or enzyme inhibition altering a drug's rate of metabolism. OTC drugs inhibiting metabolism include cimetidine and fluconazole;

Chelation by multivalent metal ions. Important examples include chelation of tetracycline or ciprofloxacin by multivalent metal ions, which can lead to treatment failure. OTC antacids and mineral supplements are the most likely culprits;

Additive, antagonistic, or synergistic effects through common end-response. Sedative antihistamines and other central nervous system depressants can worsen drowsiness and cause accidents or falls, particular among elderly people[3]; *and*

Synergistic actions on the kidney, eg, when patients taking angiotensin-converting-enzyme inhibitors take OTC aspirin or ibuprofen. Renal effects can also alter excretion of a drug or product, eg, high-potassium, low-sodium salt substitutes are potentially dangerous in patients taking potassium-sparing diuretic agents.

Homoeopathic and herbal remedies

In theory, the concentration of any purported active agent in homoeopathic products is so low that clinically significant interactions are unlikely. However, adulterants present in unlicensed products may lead to interactions[4]. As the composition and the pharmacological activities of most herbal and traditional ethnic remedies are poorly defined, interactions with such products are, on the whole, unpredictable. There are reports of interactions with conventional agents adulterating such products, eg, salicylates and non-steroidal anti-inflammatory agents. Karela, a traditional Indian medicine, may cause hypoglycaemia in diabetic patients taking insulin or sulphonylureas.

Foodstuffs, including grapefruit juice (which contains a potent enzyme inhibitor), and alcohol can also cause problems.

Assessing potential severity

One of the major difficulties in the evaluation of a potential drug interaction, and hence the course of action to adopt when faced with it, is assessing whether it is likely to lead to clinically significant adverse effects. Most drug interactions are identified on the basis of case reports or on their pharmacological plausibility. However, experimental results may not be clinically relevant.

The dosage and pack-size of an OTC product may be limited, but there is less control over its use than that of a prescription product, so such limits are no guarantee of safety. Proper labelling and packaging should minimise the risk but patients do not always read product labels, or choose to disregard the warnings. A patient who has previously had a product on prescription might follow the same pattern of use after buying it OTC.

Sources of information

Readily available and useful sources of information on drug interactions include Appendix 1 of the British National Formulary, the Compendium of data sheets and summary of product characteristics, and the monthly

Table 1: *Some potentially serious adverse drug reactions between OTC and prescribed medicines*

OTC product	Prescribed drugs	Outcome
_A-D_		
Antacids	Ciprofloxacin, tetracycline	Impaired absorption, possible treatment failure
Antihistamines, sedating	CNS depressants, eg diazepam	Increased sedation
Aspirin	Alcohol	Increased risk of gastritis
	Methotrexate	Increased risk of renal toxicity
	NSAIDs	Increased risk of gastrointestinal haemorrhage
	Warfarin	Increased risk of bleeding
Chloroquine	Cyclosporin	Increased risk of toxicity
	Methotrexate	Increased risk of nephrotoxicity
	Warfarin	Increased risk of bleeding
Cimetidine	Amiodarone, flecainide	Increased concentration and risk of adverse effects
	Phenytoin	Anticonvulsant toxicity
	Procainamide, quinidine	Increased concentration and risk of adverse effects
	Warfarin	Increased INR and risk of bleeding
Domperidone	Bromocryptine, cabergoline	Inhibition of hypoprolactinaemic effects

NSAID = Non steroidal anti-inflammatory drug

Fluconazole	Astemizole, cisapride, terfenadine	Increased risk of toxicity
	Low dose oral contraceptives	Possible increased risk of contraceptive failure
Ibuprofen	Cyclosporin, tacrolimus	Possible enhanced nephrotoxicity
	Lithium	Increased serum lithium concentration
	Methotrexate	Possible enhanced toxicity
Miconazole (inc. oral gel)	Astemizole, cisapride, terfenadine	Potentially increased risk of cardiotoxicity
Paracetamol	Co-codamol, co-dydramol, co-proxamol, other products containing paracetamol	Overdosage
Paracetamol (regular, repeated dosing)	Warfarin	Possible increase in INR and bleeding
Potassium citrate	ACE-inhibitors, cyclosporin, potassium-sparing diuretics	Increased risk of hyperkalaemia
Sympathomimetic agents (ephedrine, isometheptine, phenylephrine, phenylpropanolamine pseudoephedrine)	Adrenergic neurone blockers	Reduced hypotensive effect
	Bromocriptine	Increased risk of toxicity
	MAOIs	Hypertensive crises
Theophylline	Calcium-channel blockers	Increased risk of theophylline toxicity
	Quinolone antibiotics	Increased risk of theophylline toxicity

ACE = Angiotensin-converting-enzyme, MAOI = Monoamine oxidase inhibitor,

index of medical specialities (MIMS). However, these sources are inconsistent and, individually, incomplete. In many instances of potential drug interactions, personal professional judgement will be necessary. Specialist text-books are available[5,6,7] but are less accessible.

What can doctors and pharmacists do to prevent serious interactions with OTC medicines?

The risks of serious interactions are greatest for that small number of drugs mentioned above which are used long-term and which have a narrow therapeutic index. It is prudent to warn patients who are prescribed such drugs of the need to avoid OTC drugs unless a pharmacist or doctor has checked that interactions are unlikely. For patients taking warfarin, the information is contained in the standard warfarin card.

Potential interactions can often be avoided. For this to be possible, doctors need to know which OTC medications their patients are taking. Pharmacists, on the other hand, need to know which prescribed medications are being taken by patients. Patient records held by both doctors and pharmacists are incomplete in this respect. In the hustle and bustle of everyday clinical practice, this information gap may lead to serious consequences and vigilance is necessary by all concerned, including the patient.

Adverse effects from any OTC product, including adverse drug interactions, are reported to the Committee on Safety of Medicines (CSM) on a 'Yellow Card' in the same way as any other adverse drug reaction. Since the nature and incidence of adverse effects is less well established for OTC drugs, such reports are particularly valuable.

Conclusions

- OTC medications can interact with many prescribed drugs.
- Herbal and 'traditional' medicines pose a special problem, since their ingredients are often not well characterised.

- Most of those interactions are unlikely to have major consequences, but a few are potentially lethal.
- Patients taking prescription drugs which have a low therapeutic index, particularly warfarin, should be warned of the potential danger of interaction with OTC medicines.
- Doctors and pharmacists who suspect an adverse drug interaction or reaction involving an OTC medicine should report it to the CSM via the Yellow Card Scheme.

References
1. Honig PK, Gillespie BK. Drug interactions between prescribed and over-the-counter medication. *Drug Saf* 1995; **13:** 296-303.
2. Bailey DG, Malcolm J, Arnold O, Spence JD. Grapefruit juice-drug interactions. *Br J Clin Pharmacol* 1998; **46:** 101-10.
3. Anonymous. Alcohol warning on over-the-counter pain medications. *WHO Drug Information* 1998; **12:** 16.
4. Chan TY. Drug interactions as a cause of overanticoagulation and bleedings in Chinese patients receiving warfarin. *Int J Clin Pharmacol Ther* 1998; **36:** 403-5.
5. Hansten PD. *Drug interactions.* Baltimore: Lippincott Williams and Wilkins, 1998.
6. Stockley I. *Drug interactions.* London: Pharmaceutical Press, 1999.
7. The Medical Letter on Drugs and Therapeutics Handbook of Adverse Drug Interactions. 1998, Medical Letter Inc.

Correspondence

Community-acquired pneumonia (Volume 39 Number 2, p81)

To the Editor:

I would be interested in the authors' comments on their statement "adequate hydration and bed rest are essential", in view of the writings of Asher[1] on the dangers of bed rest.

The Surgery   **Michael G Bamber**
Back Lane
Colsterworth
Grantham
Lincs NG33 5NJ

Reference
1. Richard Asher talking sense. 1992, British Medical Association.

To the Editor:

This article includes erythromycin for empirical therapy of mild community-acquired pneumonia. This drug is poorly tolerated, with some patients experiencing nausea, vomiting and abdominal discomfort. Specific suggestions to use enteric-coated erythromycin capsules may be more useful. The newer macrolides, eg, azithromycin and clarithromycin are well tolerated with little gastrointestinal disturbance and their minimum inhibitory concentrations (MICs) against the common pathogens causing atypical pneumonia are comparable to erythromycin[1].

The article also suggests that a third-generation cephalosporin be included in the treatment of severe pneumonia. And, although this is part of the regimen suggested by the British Thoracic Society, there is a high incidence of *Clostridium difficile* diarrhoea induced by widespread empirical use of these drugs, particularly on geriatric units[2,3]. In one unit where this was a problem, the protocol was changed to a combination of clarithromycin, penicillin and ciprofloxacin without any noted difference in efficacy[3].

Senior Registrar Medical Microbiology   **GM Viagappan**
St George's Hospital
London SW17 0QT

Consultant Microbiologist   **PYC Lee**
North Middlesex Hospital
London N18 1QX

References
1. O'Grady F, Lambert HP, Finch RG, et al. Antibiotic and Chemotherapy. Churchill Livingstone 1997.
2. Impallomeni M, Galletly NP, Wort SJ, et al. Increased risk of diarrhoea caused by *Clostridium difficile* in elderly patients receiving cefotaxime. *BMJ* 1995; **311:** 1345-6.
3. Golledge CL, McKenzie T, Riley T. Extended spectrum cephalosporins and *Clostridium difficile*. *J Antimicrob Chemother* 1989; **23:** 929-31.

Authors' reply
We would like to emphasise that adequate hydration is very important in patients with community-acquired pneumonia, otherwise sputum retention may be exacerbated. As many patients, including some of those managed in the community with be hypoxic in the acute stage, rest would seem to be prudent although we are – of course – not advocating a return to the 'bad old days' of prolonged bed rest and subsequent risk of complications such as venous thrombosis. We would certainly recommend early mobilisation of patients responding to treatment for community-acquired pneumonia.

We agree that oral eryrthromycin is often poorly tolerated and that enteric-coated formulations may improve compliance; alternatively, clarithromycin is effective, with a lower incidence of gastrointestinal side-effects. We have some concerns about azithromycin as blood levels of this antibiotic are very low, which would be of concern in patients with potential bacteraemia. We agree that some cephalosporins have been linked to an increased incidence of *Clostridium difficile* diarrhoea and support the suggestion that alternative antibiotic regimens should be used where it has become a significant problem.

Department of Respiratory Medicine   **David Honeybourne**
Birmingham Heartlands Hospital   **Omer Khair**
Birmingham B9 5SS

Choice of non-steroidal anti-inflammatory drug (Volume 39 Number 2, p102)

To the Editor:
This article did not adequately address the potential hazard of non-steroidal anti-inflammatory drug (NSAID) co-administration with other drugs (besides anticoagulants), which is particularly important in patients with hypertension and diabetes mellitus.

Hyperkalaemia and renal impairment are serious adverse effects of angiotensin-converting-enzyme (ACE) inhibitors[1]. The co-administration of an NSAID could potentially worsen these adverse effects in patients treated with ACE inhibitors, possible with a fatal outcome. Furthermore, the addition of an NSAID may reduce the antihypertensive effects of ACE inhibitors[2].

Lactic acidosis is a serious complication of metformin therapy, with a mortality of 50%[3]. It tends to occur predominantly in patients with renal failure as metformin is exclusively excreted by the kidneys[3]. NSAIDs could precipitate acute renal failure in susceptible individuals, resulting in metformin-associated lactic acidosis[4], which is particularly important in patients with diabetes mellitus who may already have underlying renal complications eg, diabetic nephropathy and renal vascular disease.

Pharmacovigilance is important when prescribing NSAIDs for patients already receiving ACE inhibitors and metformin, with regular electrolyte and renal function monitoring. Also, there should be a caution on the package insert of NSAIDs bought over-the-counter.

University College London Medical School   **Norman Chan**
Department of Epidemiology & Public Health
British Heart Foundation Research Fellow
London WC1E 6BT

References
1. Chan NN, Feher MD. Long-term ACE inhibitor therapy in diabetic nephropathy: potential hazard? *Diabetic Medicine* 1998; **15:** 524.
2. Johnson AG. NSAIDs and increased blood pressure. What is the clinical significance? *Drug Saft* 1997; **17(5):** 277-89.
3. Chan NN, Brain HPS, Feher MD. Metformin-associated lactic acidosis: a rare or very rare clinical entity? *Diabetic Medicine* 1999; **16(4):** 273-81.
4. Chan NN, Fauvel NJ, Feher MD. NSAID and metformin: a cause for concern? *Lancet* 1998; **352:** 201.

To the Editor:
This article lists a wide range of adverse effects that have been described, focusing principally on the gastrointestinal tract, skin, renal tract and liver. I am, however, concerned that it recommends that NSAIDs should be avoided, or used with extreme caution, in patients with hypersensitivity reactions, including aspirin-induced asthma but not all asthma.

While working at a health authority, I had to refer to the *British National Formulary* (*BNF*) following a complaint received from a patient who had been rushed to the Accident and Emergency Department of the local general hospital with acute asthma following ingestion of prescribed ibuprofen. The patient's asthma was not known to be aspirin-induced. The *BNF* states that NSAIDs are contraindicated in patients with hypersensitivity to them, including those whose asthma has been precipitated by aspirin or another NSAID. It also carries a warning from the Committee on Safety of Medicines (CSM) that any degree of worsening of asthma may be related to ingestion of NSAIDs.

Senior Registrar   **Olatokunbo Sangowawa**
Department of Epidemiology
 & Public Health
University of Newcastle NE2 4HH

Author's response
Concerning interactions between NSAIDs and other drugs we noted that all NSAIDs can cause fluid retention, reduce the efficacy of diuretics and hypertensives and 'precipitate heart failure'. We also noted that inhibition of renal artery prostaglandin synthesis occurs and can cause deterioration of renal function. We did not go into specific interactions with individual drugs because of limitations of space, and also because the title of the article was Choice of NSAID. Appendix 1 of the BNF gives an excellent summary and prescribers should consult it. However, we are grateful to Dr Chan for drawing attention to the severity of potential interactions, particularly with metformin. What is not clear is how important, in terms of frequency such interactions are, as a literature search revealed only three cases reported to CSM.

We agree with Dr Sangowawa about patients with asthma, but the remit of our article was to discuss the choice.

Rheumatology and Rehabilitation Research Unit   **Paul Emery**
School of Medicine
University of Leeds
Leeds LS2 9NZ

Answers to correspondents

Leg ulcer management

I am currently treating a difficult venous leg ulcer in an elderly female patient and found the article by Cooke and Nicolaides on management of leg ulcers (Volume 37 Number 2, p61) most helpful. However, I wonder whether there is a place for local application of antibiotics to control bacterial overgrowth and promote healing, and what the role of microbiology in determining sensitivities as a choice factor in local antibiotic applications might be.

I would be interested to learn whether sensitivities are routinely or occasionally used in local antibiotic choice. It would also be interesting to know whether some doctors still use antiseptic preparations such as chlorhexidine acetate tulle gras dressing.

Campshill Surgery   **William Lettington**
Campshill Road
London SE13 6QU

Replies:
Bacterial overgrowth of leg ulcers is usually a mixed growth of coliforms and anaerobes which, on the whole, does not require treatment. They can produce rather smelly discharges, which we find may helpfully be controlled with topical metronidazole gel or, occasionally, topical silver sulphadiazine. The same improvement can sometimes be achieved simply with a change of dressing or an alteration in the compression bandaging regime. Personally, I do not like using topical antiseptic preparations on leg ulcers, or, indeed, topical

antibiotics (with the above exceptions), primarily because of the high risk of contact sensitivity and subsequent dermatitis.

Consultant Dermatologist   **Paul M Collier**
Royal Devon & Exeter Hospital (Wonford)
Exeter EX2 5DW

Venous leg ulcers are colonised with a variety of micro-organisms including aerobic organisms and facultative and obligate anaerobes. The latter are found deep in the base of the ulcer, when present. As superficial swabs will yield only colonising organisms, which are of little relevance to the pathogenesis of the ulcer, they are at best unhelpful in management and, at worse, misleading.

If a truly representative picture is required, a biopsy of the ulcer edge or a deep swab beneath the superficial slough is required. Infecting (as opposed to colonising) organisms will lead to cellulitis. Relevant organisms will be *Staphylococcus aureus*, beta-haemolytic streptococci, and obligate anaerobes, and their presence requires systemic therapy with appropriate antibiotics. Topical antibiotics should not be used; the ulcer will not be sterilised, but will become colonised with resistant organisms. For this reason we do not report routinely the antibiotic sensitivities of organisms isolated from superficial ulcer swabs.

If a reduction in bacterial load is required, topical disinfectants such as chlorhexidine cream may be used. Silver sulphadiazine will be effective against *Pseudomonas aeruginosa*, but resistance will develop with prolonged use. Metronidazole cream does have a role in the reduction of anearobic flora (and therefore unpleasant odour), I indolent and malignant ulcers, but has not activity against *Pseudomonas aeruginosa*. Debridement with sterile saline is a better method of reducing bacterial load.

Consultant Microbiologist   **Geoffrey Ridgway**
University College Hospital
London WC1E 6DB

INDEX

1997-99 Volumes 37 to 39

Note: alphabetisation is word-by-word, for example calcium-channel
before calcium antagonists, cod liver before codeine.

A

B

H

K

L

Q

R

Vertigo contd.

management	1998, **38,** 93-6
prevalence	1998, **38,** 87
symptoms	1998, **38,** 90-
Vigabatrin for epilepsy	1998, **38,** 99-101
Vinca alkaloids causing intestinal distension	1997, **37,** 191
Vincristine for chronic lymphocytic leukaemia	1998, **38,** 22,23
see also Vinca alkaloids	
Vitamin B12 deficiency and supplementation	1997, **37,** 88
Vitamin D for osteoporosis	1997, **37,** 117
Vomiting in terminal illness	1998, **38,** 33
see also Nausea and vomiting	

W

Warfarin	
in atrial fibrillation	1997, **37,** 173
in elderly patients	1998, **38,** 230
in pulmonary hypertension	1998, **38,** 163
indications	1997, **37,** 173
initiation	1997, **37,** 174
interactions	1997, **37,** 177-78
maintenance dosage	1997, **37,** 176
mechanism of action	1997, **37,** 173
monitoring	1997, **37,** 176
prescribing	1997, **37,** 173,177
stopping treatment	1997, **37,** 177
Watchful waiting	
for symptomless localised prostatic cancer	1999, **39,** 18
White-coat hypertension *see* Hypertension, white-coat	
White soft paraffin for crab louse infestation	1998, **38,** 82
Withdrawal of antihypertensive drugs	
advantages	1997, **37,** 146
patient identification	1997, **37,** 147
problems	1997, **37,** 149
studies	1997, **37,** 146
Wound	
assessment and evaluation	1998, **38,** 116-7
infection control	1998, **38,** 119
management	1998, **38,** 117-21

Y

Z